Neurological Emergencies

Neurological Emergencies

S.D. Shorvon MB, BChir, MA, MD, MRCP

Senior lecturer in Neurology and Honorary Consultant Neurologist, Institute of Neurology and National Hospital for Nervous Diseases, London, and National Hospital/Chalfont Centre for Epilepsy, Chalfont St Peter, Buckinghamshire.

Butterworths
London, Boston, Singapore, Sydney, Toronto, Wellington

in association with
Current Medical Literature Ltd.
London

PART OF REED INTERNATIONAL P.L.C.

All rights reserved. No part of this publication may be reproduced or transmitted in any form or by any means (including photocopying and recording) without the written permission of the copyright holder except in accordance with the provisions of the Copyright Act 1956 (as amended) or under the terms of a licence issued by the Copyright Licensing Agency Ltd, 33–34 Alfred Place, London, England WC1E 7DP. The written permission of the copyright holder must also be obtained before any part of this publication is stored in a retrieval system of any nature. Applications for the copyright holder's written permission to reproduce, transmit or store in a retrieval system any part of this publication should be addressed to the Publishers.

Warning: The doing of an unauthorised act in relation to a copyright work may result in both a civil claim for damages and criminal prosecution.

This book is sold subject to the Standard Conditions of Sale of Net Books and may not be re-sold in the UK below the net price given by the Publishers in the current price list.

First published 1989

© **Current Medical Literature Ltd 1989**

British Library Cataloguing in Publication Data

Shorvon, S. D.
  Neurological emergencies.
  1. Man. Nervous system. Diseases &
  injuries. Emergency treatment
  I. Title
  616.8'0425

ISBN 0-407-00873-X

Library of Congress Cataloging in Publication Data

Shorvon, S. D. (Simon D.)
  Neurological emergencies.

  Includes bibliographies and index.
  1. Central nervous system--Diseases. 2. Medical
emergencies. I. Title. [DNLM: 1. Emergencies.
2. Nervous System Diseases. WL 100 S559n]
RC361.S46   1989   616.8'0425   88-26278
ISBN 0-407-00873-X

Printed in Great Britain at the University Press, Cambridge

Contents

Preface

1. Coma

Causes
    Focal supratentorial lesion
    Focal subtentorial lesion
    Diffuse neurological or systemic disturbance
Emergency management
    Emergency resuscitation
    Initial diagnostic assessment
        History
        General examination
        Circulation (pulse and blood pressure)
        Neurological examination
        Emergency investigations
    Serial monitoring
    Emergency treatment
        Glucose
        Thiamine
        Increased intracranial pressure
        Seizures
        Hypothermia/hyperthermia
        Acid-base balance
        Metabolic disturbance
        Infection
        Transtentorial herniation (coning)
        Specific measures
        Other measures
        Neurological/neurosurgical referral
Transtentorial herniation (tentorial coning)
Further reading

2. Acute Infective Encephalitis

Acute viral encephalitis
    Emergency treatment
        Admission to hospital
        Stupor/coma
        Raised intracranial pressure
        Seizures
        Specific antiviral therapy
Non-viral infective encephalitis
Further reading

3. Meningitis

Viral meningitis
    Clinical features
    Laboratory findings
    Treatment
Bacterial meningitis
    Clinical features
    Laboratory findings
    Emergency Treatment
        Antibiotic treatment
        Other treatment
    Problems in diagnosis and management
        Optic disc changes suggesting raised intracranial pressure
        Focal neurological signs or coma
        Partially treated meningitis
        Sterile meningitis
        Recurrent meningitis
        Neonatal meningitis
        Tuberculous meningitis
Other forms of infective meningitis
    Fungal meningitis
    Meningovascular syphilis
    Other
Further reading

4. Intracranial Abscess and Venous Thrombosis/Thrombophlebitis

Cerebral abscess
    Clinical features
    Investigations
        CT
        Lumbar puncture
        Cerebral angiography/EEG
        Culture/haematology/biochemistry
        Other
    Emergency treatment
Intracranial subdural empyema
    Clinical features
    Diagnosis
    Emergency treatment
Intracranial extradural abscess
Cerebral venous thrombosis/thrombophlebitis
    Cortical vein thrombosis/thrombophlebitis
    Cavernous sinus thrombosis/thrombophlebitis
    Diagnosis
    Investigations
    Emergency treatment
        Establish/treat underlying cause
        Seizures
        Other

5. Stroke and Subarachnoid Haemorrhage

Stroke
    Diagnosis
        Differentiation between haemorrhage and infarction
        Identification of the site of damage
        Identification of the underlying cause
    Emergency investigations
        General investigations
        CT and skull X-ray
        Cerebral angiography

　　　　Lumbar puncture
　　　Emergency management
　　　　Anticoagulants
　　　　Antihypertensive agents
　　　　Emergency surgery
　　　　General measures
Subarachnoid haemorrhage
　　　Diagnosis
　　　Emergency investigations
　　　Emergency management
　　　　General measures
　　　　Prevention of further haemorrhage
Further reading

6. Head Injury

Initial assessment
Admission to hospital
Early hospital management
　　　The unconscious patient
　　　The conscious patient
　　　Transfer to or consultation with neurosurgical department
Immediate complications
　　　Laceration and open head injury
　　　Linear skull fracture
　　　Depressed skull fracture
　　　Acute extradural haemorrhage
　　　Acute subdural haemorrhage
　　　Acute intracerebral haemorrhage
　　　Post-traumatic seizures
　　　Cranial nerve injury
　　　Inappropriate ADH secretion
　　　Other injury
Further reading

7. Acute Spinal Cord Dysfunction

Clinical features of spinal cord dysfunction
    Spinal pain
    Motor signs
    Sensory signs
    Sphincteric signs
    Respiratory signs
Acute spinal cord compression
    Metastatic tumour
    Primary tumour
    Infection
    Disc disease
    Degenerative spinal column disease
    Epidural haematoma
Acute non-compressive spinal cord lesions
    Acute transverse myelitis
    Vascular infarction
    Cervical spondylosis
    Other causes
Emergency management in acute spinal cord dysfunction
Acute spinal cord injury
    Emergency assessment
        Neurological
        Orthopaedic
        Respiratory function
    Movement of the patient
    Radiological diagnosis
    Other measures
    Other complications
    Treatment

8. Status Epilepticus

Emergency management
    Resuscitation
        IV line

Protection of cardiorespiratory function
Thiamine and glucose
Emergency investigations
Aetiology and precipitating factors
Medical complications
Anticonvulsant therapy
Immediate seizure control
Long-term seizure control
Intramuscular drug administration
Refractory status epilepticus
Drug treatment of status epilepticus in children
Further reading

9. Acute Respiratory Failure Due to Neurological Disease

Diagnosis
Respiratory failure
Underlying neurological disease
Emergency management
Immediate assessment of ventilation
Other measures
Investigations

10. Brain Death

Aetiology
Evaluation of clinical neurological status
EEG
Other
Further reading

Index

Preface

About 10% of all emergency medical admissions are due to neurological disease. Neurology has a reputation for being complex and esoteric, yet in emergency settings this is unjustified. A simple logical approach will allow rapid diagnosis and effective treatment in the great majority of cases. Nevertheless, neurological emergencies are frequently mishandled, and this is unfortunate, as delayed diagnosis or treatment may have grave consequences for prognosis.

In this book the initial assessment and early treatment of patients presenting with neurological emergencies are outlined. The emphasis is on those clinical features that assist rapid diagnosis, emergency investigations and early treatment, and those situations in which urgent neurological or neurosurgical referral is advisable. The commonest emergencies only have been covered, and this text is no substitute for the comprehensive textbooks of neurology and therapeutics; rather it is intended as an essentially practical guide.

The book is aimed principally at the non-specialists who first receive the patient — the general practitioner, casualty officer and general medical teams — and the neurologist or neurosurgeon in training. It is often these doctors who have the burden of responsiblity for correct early management, and whose actions may profoundly affect the outcome. It is hoped that the book will make their task easier, and their practice more proficient.

S.D. Shorvon

1. Coma

Coma is one of the most common neurological emergencies in general hospital practice, and one in which skilful management may be life-saving. Four basic principles are involved: *resuscitation, diagnosis, serial monitoring* and *treatment*.

Resuscitation is directed primarily at ensuring adequate circulatory and respiratory function. Diagnosis may seem daunting, as almost any intrinsic or extrinsic malfunction of the upper brain stem or extensive bilateral cerebral disorder can lead to coma, and the causes are multitudinous (Table 1.1). However, a history and careful clinical examination are usually sufficient, and these are often best carried out in the casualty or emergency room. Serial monitoring of coma is necessary to detect improvement or deterioration in clinical status, as subsequent treatment may depend as much on such changes as on the underlying pathology. Observations are best made using an objective clinical scale such as the well-tried Glasgow Coma Scale, which is based on assessment of three aspects of neurological function (Table 1.2). Emergency treatment includes both specific and non-specific therapy, which is often initiated before the precise cause of the coma has been established. Transtentorial herniation (coning) is a particular danger of supratentorial mass lesions, and the emergency physician should be aware of the signs of this serious development and its treatment.

Only conditions presenting primarily as coma are considered here although, of course, all medical illnesses may result in terminal coma. However, in such cases the non-neurological cause is usually obvious. Similarly, the management of the underlying causes in metabolic coma (e.g. diabetic coma) is not discussed in detail.

2 Coma

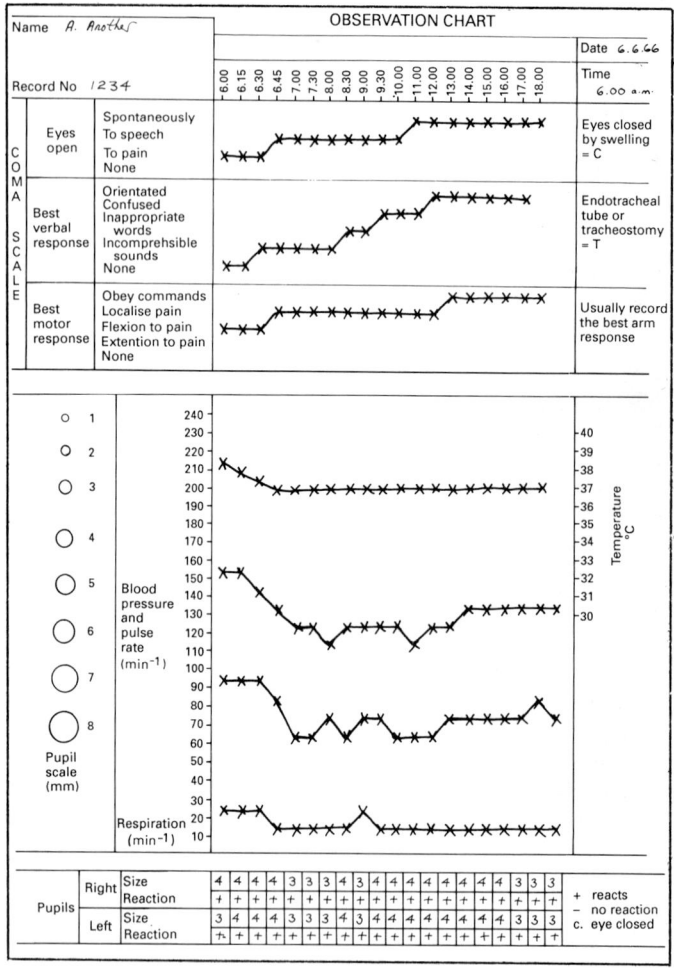

Figure 1.1 Serial monitoring chart, filled in for 12 h, of a patient making an uncomplicated recovery from coma due to head injury.

CAUSES

Diagnosis should proceed in two stages. First, the site of the neurological lesion should be identified (i.e. focal supratentorial, focal subtentorial, diffuse or systemic) and then its likely aetiology established. The conditions that present most commonly as coma at a general hospital are listed in Table 1.1.

Table 1.1 Possible causes of coma of unknown aetiology

Focal supratentorial lesions (30%)[*]
Infarction
  arterial (embolic, thrombotic, occlusive)
  venous
Haemorrhage
  intracerebral (e.g. arteriovenous malformation, hypertensive, other)
  subdural
  extradural
  secondary to subarachnoid haemorrhage
Tumour
  primary
  secondary
Abscess
  intracerebral
  extradural
  subdural
Other (e.g. hydrocephalus)

Focal subtentorial lesions (10%)[*]
Infarction
  cerebellar
  brain-stem
Haemorrhage
  cerebellar
  brain-stem
  extradural
  subdural
Tumour
  primary
  secondary
Other brain-stem disorders (e.g. abscess, aneurysm, demyelination)

Diffuse central and/or systemic disorders (60%)[*]
Diffuse neurological disorders
  epileptic seizures
  meningitis
  encephalitis
  hypoxic brain damage

subarachnoid haemorrhage
bilateral infarction
Head injury/cerebral contusion
other (e.g. cerebral malaria, pituitary apoplexy)
Systemic disturbance
diabetes (hypo/hyperglycaemia, lactic/ketotic acidosis)
renal failure
hepatic failure
hypertensive encephalopathy
hypo/hyperthermia
hypothyroidism
Addisonian crisis
Hypo/hypernatraemia
Drugs and poisoning
sedative and psychotropic drugs
alcohol
illegal drug abuse
other poisons

*Percentages refer to approx. incidence in hospital practice.

FOCAL SUPRATENTORIAL LESION

Coma develops only if the lesion is large or rapidly expanding, thereby causing secondary brain-stem compression (transtentorial coning — see below) and the prognosis is therefore poor. Papilloedema, contralateral neurological motor signs and/or conjugate deviation of the eyes towards the side of the lesion may be associated with coma in such cases, and are valuable localizing signs. The initial signs are usually those of focal hemispheric disease (e.g. asymmetrical motor signs) and the signs of deteriorating function usually progress caudally.

FOCAL SUBTENTORIAL LESION

Alteration of consciousness may be abrupt, or may proceed from other brain-stem signs. Breathing patterns are often bizarre and signs of localized brain-stem disturbance (e.g. dysconjugate oculomotor disturbance (positional or reflex), skew deviation, cranial nerve palsy) may be prominent. Sometimes such signs are mimicked by supratentorial disease causing brain-stem compression, but in such cases these are usually late signs. Both conjugate eye deviation and hemiparesis may be caused by supratentorial or subtentorial disease; in the former the eyes are usually deviated towards the side of the cerebral lesion, and the contralateral hemiparesis may be accompanied by contralateral cranial nerve signs (e.g. facial weakness). Conversely, in subtentorial disease the conjugate deviation is often away from the side of the lesion, and the cranial nerve signs are contralateral to the limb weakness (crossed hemiplegia).

DIFFUSE NEUROLOGICAL OR SYSTEMIC DISTURBANCE

If diffuse supratentorial disease (without transtentorial herniation) causes coma, the cerebral disorder must be bilateral and widespread; hence coma often denotes a poor prognosis. The history or the temporal progression of the condition may often make the aetiology clear, and clinical signs vary depending on the underlying cause. In strictly supratentorial disease, however, brain-stem function will be preserved even in deep coma.

In systemic disease coma is due to diffuse, often reversible, brain dysfunction. The onset is often gradual, and confusion or stupor may precede coma. In contrast to focal brain disease, focal neurological signs are entirely absent, motor signs are symmetrical, reflex brain-stem functions (e.g. reflex eye movement, blink reflex) are usually present and limb signs (e.g. flaccidity, reflex changes) are usually symmetrical. In deep coma (e.g. due to drug intoxication) brain-stem reflexes may be abolished, but pupillary reflexes are usually present unless the drug acts directly on the pupil, as do opiates. Characteristically, in metabolic coma signs may fluctuate and seem inconsistent, with some functions preserved and others lost (e.g. a preserved corneal response but absent reflex eye movements). The EEG is often helpful in assessing metabolic coma, and the CT scan will be normal. Tremor, asterixis, myoclonus and seizures are common in stuporose and comatose patients with metabolic disorders, but both myoclonus and seizures may also occur in structural cerebral disease. The commonest causes of coma in the UK fall into this category, and include drug and alcohol overdose, head injury, and diabetic coma.

EMERGENCY MANAGEMENT

EMERGENCY RESUSCITATION

The first priority is to safeguard cardiorespiratory function. In the absence of co-existent cardiovascular disease, this is threatened only in deep coma. Pulse, blood pressure and respiratory rate should be measured, the airways protected and the patient kept in the 'coma position' (Fig 1.2). If there is any evidence of respiratory insufficiency, artificial respiration should be considered; it is better to institute this early rather than late in the development of respiratory failure (here management differs from that of cardiorespiratory disease). If there is co-existent spinal injury, care should be taken not to extend the neck while intubating the patient. A secure IV line should be introduced into a large vein and IV fluid-replacement therapy initiated.

INITIAL DIAGNOSTIC ASSESSMENT

History
The history may be diagnostic, but it is surprising how often this simple fact is ignored. Questioning the relatives,

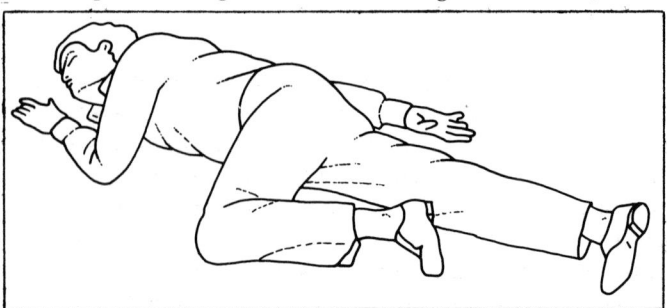

Figure 1.2 The coma position, with the patient semi-prone, to minimize the danger of airway obstruction or inhalation of vomit.

passers-by, ambulance drivers, etc. may help establish the cause of the coma (e.g. they may report finding insulin, empty tablet bottles, or signs of alcoholism).

General examination

General examination of the patient may reveal a Medi-Alert bracelet, gum hypertrophy due to phenytoin, signs of drug abuse or of injury, meningism or other signs of CNS infection, blood in the ear (in cases of skull fracture), jaundice or ketosis. Co-existent non-neurological disorders, including traumatic damage, burns or pressure sores, should be carefully identified and documented. These may need emergency treatment in their own right. Direct injury to the eye (or oculomotor nerves) may also complicate the neurological assessment.

Circulation (pulse and blood pressure)

Abnormalities of pulse and blood pressure are usually a late and ominous sign in coma, especially if due to structural damage. In severe metabolic coma, however, hypotension is often noted. In trauma a more common cause of hypotension is blood loss due to co-existing injury, and it is easy to overlook this in a comatose patient.

Neurological examination

This is important both in the determination of the site of dysfunction and in establishing a base-line for further monitoring. In a comatose patient the following aspects should be covered.

Level of consciousness: this is a vital measurement, and yet it is surprising to see how often it is ignored. The most simple, well standardised and effective method of recording this is to use the Glasgow Coma Scale (Table 1.2). As responses may fluctuate, the best response elicited at each examination should be recorded. In assessing verbal response, confused speech is defined as conversation with correct syntax but confused content; 'inappropriate words' means intelligible but isolated words. Motor responses should be tested in all four limbs. If command elicits no

Table 1.2 Glasgow Coma Scale

Score	Eye opening	Best verbal response	Best motor response
5		orientated	obeys commands
4	spontaneous	confused	localizes to painful stimuli
3	to speech	inappropriate words	flexion movements to painful stimuli
2	to painful stimuli	incomprehensible sounds	extension movement to painful stimuli
1	never	none	none

response, gentle but sustained painful stimuli should be applied to each extremity and to the supraorbital notch.

Respiration: the respiratory rate should be recorded. The respiratory pattern (Fig 1.3) should be assessed and recorded as regular, periodic (e.g. Cheyne-Stokes) or ataxic, and other irregularities noted. In focal hemispheric lesions the pattern may be normal or Cheyne-Stokes respiration may occur. The latter may imply bilateral and deep diencephalic or midbrain damage (although it can occur in other situations, e.g. in metabolic coma or circulatory defects). In high brain-stem dysfunction, hyperventilation may also occur. In pontine lesions respiration may be shallow or cluster. Apneustic breathing localises the area of damage to the mid or caudal pontine region. In medullary lesions respiration may be slow and irregular, gasping or ataxic. Yawning or hiccupping may also occur in brain-stem damage.

Pupils: these should be examined for size, equality and reactivity, using a strong flashlight (an eye lens may be necessary to observe reactivity). Pupil reactions are usually normal in coma due to cerebral hemisphere damage. In

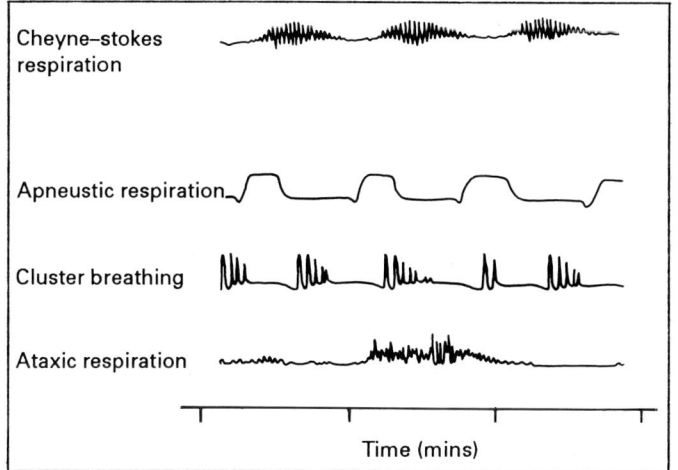

Figure 1.3 Abnormal respiratory patterns in coma. Diagnostic presentation of four abnormal respiratory paterns, from tracing from an abdominal pneumograph. Inspiration is represented by an upstroke, and expiration by a downstroke. The amplitude of the waves is proportional to the amplitude of the respiratory excursions.

lesions at the level of the midbrain they are often middle-sized and fixed; in pontine lesions they are usually pinpoint. A unilateral fixed dilated pupil is usually due to a third nerve lesion, which in coma suggests uncal coning.

Eye movements: the position at rest of the eyes and any spontaneous movement should be noted. Reflex movements should be recorded to brisk horizontal head turning (oculocephalic reflex) and to caloric stimulation with up to 50 ml of ice-cold water with the head at 30° above the horizontal plane (oculovestibular reflex) (Table 1.3). The oculocephalic reflex should not be tested if there is the possibility of a major neck injury — the eardrums should be inspected before testing the oculovestibular reflex. If asymmetrical the movement of each eye should be detailed separately. In focal cerebral hemisphere lesions there may be conjugate deviation towards the side of the lesion, there are usually no spontaneous movements although sometimes slow roving eye movements occur. The oculocephalic

10 Coma

Table 1.3 The oculocephalic and oculovestibular reflexes

Oculocephalic reflex (Doll's head manoeuvre)

This is elicited by sharply rotating the patient's head from side to side through 60°, pausing briefly at the extremes of each lateral movement.

Normal	Rotation of the head, produces conjugate deviation of the eyes in the opposite direction (i.e. if the head is rotated to the left, the eyes rotate to right), so that the patient appears to stare in a direction opposite to direction of head rotation.
Coma	In metabolic coma or coma due to diffuse or focal supratentorial disease, the reflex is usually normal unless coma is deep; in subtentorial disorders causing coma, the reflex may be lost or the eye movements may be dysconjugate.
Brain death	The reflex is lost. The eyes move with the head (and thus the patient appears to continue to stare straight ahead).

Oculovestibular reflex (caloric reflex)

This is elicited by syringing 50 mls of cold (preferably ice cold) water into each ear in turn, with the head resting at about 30° from the horizontal. Before carrying out this test, it is important to inspect the ear, to ensure that the water reaches the tympanic membrane, and to exclude ear diseases which might interfere with the reflex.

Normal	Nystagmus is induced, with the slow phase towards the side of irrigation.
Coma	In metabolic disease or supratentorial disease, the eyes become tonically deviated towards the side of the irrigation (in deep coma, the reflex may be lost altogether); in subtentorial lesions, the evoked eye movements may be disconjugate.
Brain death	The reflex is lost. No movement of the eyes is elicited.

Notes:
- If the eyes of the comatose patient are closed, they can be taped open carefully before carrying out these tests.
- Both reflexes may be depressed by sedative medication such as anticonvulsants, antidepressants, anticholinergics, neuromuscular blocking drugs, ototoxic drugs.

reflexes can usually be demonstrated and caloric testing produces tonic deviation rather than nystagmus. The reflexes are usually powerful enough to overcome any resting conjugate deviation. In metabolic coma the reflex eye movements are usually normal, even in the presence of signs of brain-stem depression (e.g. decorticate movements), although in very deep coma they may be suppressed. In midbrain or pontine lesions various abnormalities of position, spontaneous movement and reflex movement may be observed, including skew deviation, ocular palsies, ocular bobbing or conjugate deviation (vertical or horizontal) depending on the level and extent of damage. In coma dysconjugate movements (spontaneous or reflex) almost always imply brain-stem dysfunction. As a rule of thumb if the eyes are conjugately deviated at rest and cannot be brought past the midline by reflex testing, the lesion is usually pontine. Conjugate deviation correctable past the midline by reflex testing implies a hemisphere lesion.

Motor function: the motor response (as on the Glasgow Coma Scale) should be recorded, as should the limb tone and reflexes. Loss of motor function in a lightly comatose patient is demonstrated by asymmetrical responses to painful stimulation, but in a deeply comatose patient this may not be possible to elicit. Decorticate movements (flexion of the arm and extension of the leg) and decerebrate movements (extensor responses of the arms and legs) may occur spontaneously or be elicited by painful or other stimuli. The presence of decerebrate or particularly decorticate movements often carries an ominous prognosis. In focal hemisphere dysfunction the motor abnormalities are usually contralateral, although in acute massive hemisphere lesions (e.g. head injury or haemorrhage) decerebrate posturing may be due to selective depression of brain-stem function. In focal midbrain lesions the abnormalities are usually bilateral, and decorticate or decerebrate posturing may be elicited. In pontine or medullary lesions abnormalities are usually bilateral and/or symmetrical, and decerebrate posturing may be observed. In severe pontine or medullary damage there is usually no movement and tone will be flaccid.

Other neurological signs: these may give a clue to localisation or aetiology. Thus, papilloedema suggests raised intracranial pressure (usually due to a space-occupying lesion); cranial nerve palsies suggest brain-stem disease; meningism suggests meningitis or subarachnoid haemorrhage; subhyaloid haemorrhage suggests subarachnoid haemorrhage.

Emergency investigations
In all cases of coma of unknown aetiology, initial investigations should be carried out as outlined in Table 1.4.

SERIAL MONITORING
The serial monitoring of comatose patients is an essential aspect of management. Unconscious patients should be attended at all times. Vital signs and level of consciousness should be observed and charted at 15-minute intervals (Table 1.5 and Fig. 1.1) until it is certain that the patient is stable or improving, and then less frequently depending on

---

Table 1.4 Emergency investigations in cases of coma of unknown aetiology

---

Emergency venous: full blood count, glucose electrolytes, urea

Emergency urinary: ketones or glucose (if quicker than blood estimations)

Emergency arterial: blood gases, pH (repeated as necessary)

Rapid venous: liver function, calcium, osmolarity, lactate, cortisol, drug/alcohol/poison screen, culture (as required); 50 ml of serum saved for later toxicological testing and other uses

Rapid EEG: in cases of metabolic coma (and as required)

Emergency CT: in cases of structural brain disease (usually after neurosurgical/neurological referral), if intracranial pressure is raised or transtentorial coning is suspected.

Emergency LP: in some cases of meningitis

*Table 1.5 Serial clinical monitoring**

Pulse
Blood pressure
Respiratory rate
Pupillary size, reactivity, equality
Glasgow Coma Scale measurements

*To be carried out at 15-min intervals until the patient's status has stabilized or is definitely improving.

the diagnosis. Deterioration in any of these parameters should be reported immediately to the doctor in charge; it is often forgotten that this is the point of serial monitoring.

EMERGENCY TREATMENT

Glucose
In any unconscious patient in whom the diagnosis is obscure, 50 ml of 50% glucose solution should be infused via the IV line (after blood is taken for a blood glucose measure) as occult hypoglycaemia, although reversible, is potentially fatal.

Thiamine
If there is the slightest suspicion of alcoholism, 50 mg thiamine (in a preparation such as Parentrovite) should also be administered IV. This is particularly important if glucose has been administered, as Wernicke's encephalopathy may be exacerbated by glucose in the absence of thiamine.

Increased intracranial pressure
IV *corticosteroids* (dexamethasone, 4–10 mg, 6-hourly) or occasionally *mannitol* (200 ml of a 20% solution over 10 min) may be life-saving if intracranial pressure is critically increased. However, these should not be given blindly as they complicate assessment and, even in the presence of increased intracranial pressure, relief may be only temporary. Forced hyperventilation may also be used to lower intracranial pressure.

Seizures
Seizures should be treated immediately with IV anticonvulsants (Chapter 8).

Hypothermia/hyperthermia
Hypothermia (body temperature <34°C) should be corrected by cautious warming. Severe hyperthermia (often an ominous sign in comatose patients) should also be corrected immediately.

Acid-base balance
Severe metabolic acidosis or alkalosis should be corrected at a rate which depends on the cause. Slow correction may be needed in some types of metabolic coma (e.g. diabetic ketoacidosis).

Metabolic disturbance
Although a severe metabolic disturbance should also be corrected, the speed with which this is achieved will depend on the cause and the type of disturbance. Too rapid correction of hyponatraemia, for instance, may result in further neurological damage. Similarly, the management of diabetic coma depends on the level of blood glucose and associated acid-base disturbance.

Infection
As soon as samples are drawn, infection should be actively treated.

Transtentorial herniation (coning)
If this is threatened or occurring, emergency treatment should be instituted, as outlined below.

Specific measures
In certain cases of coma specific measures can be taken (e.g. IV naloxone (0.4 mg at 5 min intervals) in narcotic overdose). However, specific measures can usually be delayed until after emergency assessment and treatment.

Other measures
The eyes should be protected in a comatose patient. Skilled nursing is important also for the prevention of pressure sores.

Neurological/neurosurgical referral
Urgent neurological or neurosurgical advice should always be sought when there is:

(i) a primary neurological cause for the coma (see relevant chapters);
(ii) transtentorial herniation;
(iii) deterioration in neurological signs on serial monitoring; or
(iv) diagnosis is obscure.

TRANSTENTORIAL HERNIATION (TENTORIAL CONING)

As a supratentorial mass lesion expands, it may cause increasing compression of brain-stem structures by downward movement of the cerebral hemispheres. This is known as *transtentorial herniation* or *coning*. If the downward movement is asymmetrical, the uncus on one side may be compressed against the falx (uncal herniation) and against the ipsilateral third nerve. A more mid-line displacement will cause central herniation (Fig. 1.4). Both uncal and central herniation require immediate emergency action as irreversible brain damage may ensue, sometimes in a matter of minutes. There is sometimes a distinctive progression in clinical signs, with sequential compression of diencephalic, midbrain, pontine and then medullary functions.

If a supratentorial mass lesion is suspected as the cause of coma, arrangements should be made for immediate transfer of the patient to a neurological unit because of the danger of transtentorial herniation. Cranial CT scanning, which has revolutionized management in such cases, should be carried out as soon as possible, if necessary, while neurosurgical transfer is being arranged, even if this involves calling in

16 Coma

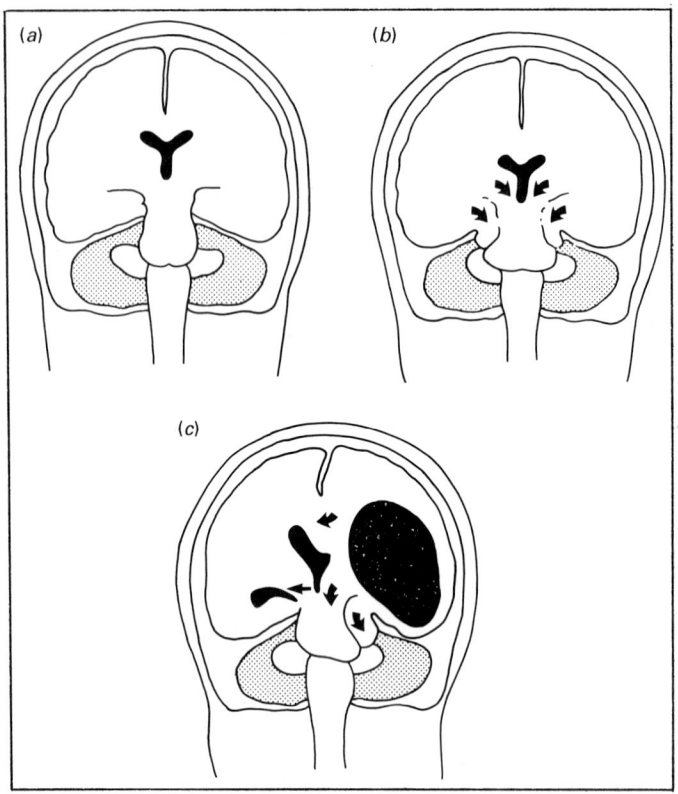

Figure 1.4 Central and uncal transtentorial herniation (coning). (a) Normal. (b) Central herniation: the diencephalon is compressed from equally distributed downward pressure. (c) Uncal herniation: the ipsilateral uncus and cingulate gyrus are pushed under the falx, and the third nerve is compressed against the edge of the falx; there is less downward displacement of the brain stem (in this example, due to a unilateral hemisphere lesion).

staff out of hours. Lumbar puncture is contraindicated in a patient with a supratentorial mass lesion (especially if it is severe enough to cause coma), as this may precipitate coning by lowering the subtentorial pressure. Unfortunately, this simple principle is frequently overlooked. If a supratentorial mass is definitely diagnosed, IV corticosteroid therapy (initially with dexamethasone, 4–10 mg, 6-hourly) should be started while awaiting neurosurgical transfer.

If coning is already occurring, or if the neurological status is deteriorating rapidly due to increasing intracranial pressure, IV mannitol should be given (200 ml of a 20% solution over 10 min), as this acts more quickly than IV steroids, although the effects are short-lived, and arrangements should be made for immediate surgical decompression. Forced hyperventilation may also temporarily lower intracranial pressure.

FURTHER READING

Plum F, Posner JB.
The Diagnosis of Stupor & Coma. Philadelphia: FA Davis & Co, 1980.
This superb monograph is the definitive work on the clinical aspects of coma.

2. Acute Infective Encephalitis

Acute intracranial infections are classified according to the site of involvement (Table 2.1). This chapter deals with the encephalitides, and the following two chapters with other forms of intracranial infection.

ACUTE VIRAL ENCEPHALITIS

Most cases of acute infective encephalitis are viral in origin; the viruses responsible for acute encephalitis in the UK are listed in Table 2.2. The most important common cause of sporadic viral encephalitis in this country is the herpes simplex type II virus. In addition to the encephalitis caused by direct invasion of nervous tissue by the virus, an immunologically based 'post-viral encephalitis' (or encephalomyelitis) can occur following viral illness or vaccination.

The clinical presentation, speed of progression and outcome of viral and post-viral encephalitis may vary greatly. At one extreme (usually due to herpes simplex infection) the disease is fulminating and frequently results in coma and death; at the other, mild headache might be the only symptom. Presenting symptoms are listed in Table 2.3. The characteristic features include fever, headache and acute changes in mental state or consciousness. Seizures are

Table 2.1 Classification of acute intracranial infections

Diffuse infection of cerebral tissue:	encephalitis
Diffuse infection of the meninges:	meningitis
Localized infection of cerebral tissue:	cerebral abscess
Localized parameningeal infection:	subdural/extradural empyema
Venous infection:	cerebral venous thrombophlebitis

Table 2.2 Causes of acute viral encephalitis in the UK

Arbovirus (e.g. louping ill)
Enterovirus (e.g. echovirus, coxsackievirus, poliovirus)
Herpesvirus (e.g. herpes simplex type II, herpes zoster)
Paramyxovirus (e.g. mumps, rubella)
Rhabdovirus (e.g. rabies)
Other (e.g. HIV, lymphocytic choriomeningitis, vaccinia)

also very common. Not surprisingly, there is frequently a meningeal element, which is usually mild, and the term meningo-encephalitis is often used. The main distinction between viral meningitis and encephalitis is that meningeal symptoms predominate in the former whereas cerebral symptoms (e.g. altered consciousness, mental changes, seizures) predominate in the latter. Specific systemic features may appear in some viral infections (e.g. parotitis in mumps, rash in exanthemata) and these may aid diagnosis, but in general it is difficult in the emergency setting to determine the causal agent. Acute viral encephalitis may also present like a cerebral abscess or tumour.

Diagnosis is usually made on the basis of clinical findings and the typical but not pathognomonic CSF changes — a lymphocytic leucocytosis (usually <500 cells/mm^3), raised

Table 2.3 Presenting clinical features of acute viral encephalitis

Headache (usually severe)
Fever, toxaemia
Altered behaviour, confusion
Depressed consciousness (e.g drowsiness, stupor, coma)
Seizures*
Meningism (usually mild)
Nausea and vomiting (uncommon)
Focal neurological signs (e.g. aphasia, hemiparesis, cranial nerve palsy)
Systemic features of specific viruses (e.g. rash, parotitis)

*Viral encephalitis may present as a single seizure, a series of seizures or as status epilepticus.
These may develop as the condition progresses, but are rare at presentation.

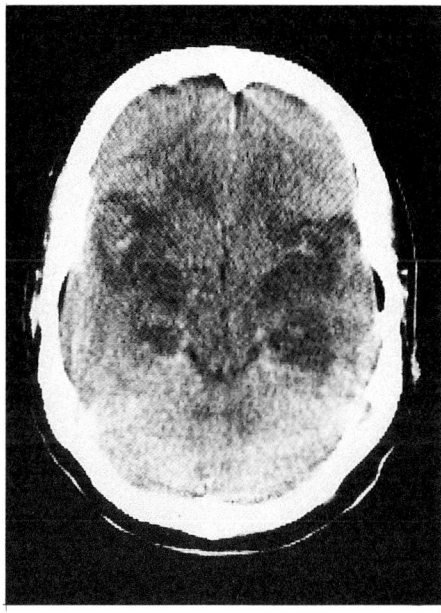

Figure 2.1 CT in acute herpes simplex encephalitis showing patchy low attenuation in both temporal regions and evidence of cerebral swelling.

protein levels (usually <200 mg/100 ml) and normal sugar levels. The virus is seldom isolated from the CSF, and exact identification may have to await immunological and serological tests. Sometimes computed tomography (CT) scanning in severe encephalitis (especially herpes simplex encephalitis) is diagnostic, showing patchy low attenuation and swelling, especially in the temporal regions (Fig 2.1). An EEG may also be helpful, usually showing generalized slowing (and occasionally more specific changes) even in mild cases and often when the CT scan is normal. However, in some cases the CSF, EEG and CT scan are normal, particularly in the early stages or in cases of mild infection. Brain biopsy has been recommended for the diagnosis of herpes simplex encephalitis, but as less toxic treatment has now become available it is no longer necessary. As there is often a meningeal component to viral encephalitis (meningo-encephalitis), it is essential to exclude bacteria and other infective agents (Chapter 3).

In most cases of viral encephalitis the diagnosis is presumptive, based as it often is on non-specific CSF, EEG or CT findings. It is therefore important to keep the diagnosis under review, and if the patient's condition does not rapidly improve on initial therapy, further CT, CSF or EEG should be carried out and alternative diagnoses considered. Of all referrals with presumed encephalitis in one big series, only 50% turned out to have encephalitis. The commonest actual diagnoses were cerebral abscess, tumour, meningitis, haemorrhage and cerebrovascular disease.

AIDS may present either as an encephalitic illness due to primary infection with the human immunodeficiency virus (HIV) (serological conversion may be seen during the course of illness) or as an encephalitis with an opportunistic infection, which is often due to unusual organisms (e.g. cytomegalovirus, toxoplasma).

EMERGENCY TREATMENT

Admission to hospital
In all but the mildest cases admission to hospital is necessary for initial observation, lumbar puncture and other investigations. Isolation is not required.

Stupor/coma
If the patient is stuporose or comatose, appropriate care must be instituted (Chapter 1).

Raised intracranial pressure
Brain swelling is a feature of many types of encephalitis. If there is clinical evidence of raised intracranial pressure, IV dexamethasone (adults: 4–10 mg, 6 hourly) should be given. Occasionally, other measures are required, such as IV mannitol infusion, hyperventilation or neurosurgical decompression, but urgent neurological advice should be sought before embarking on such measures.

Seizures
Seizures are very common and may require urgent treatment; in severe cases (when the patient is in coma) prophylactic anticonvulsant therapy with phenytoin is recommended (Chapter 8).

Specific antiviral therapy
Specific antiviral therapy with acyclovir should be started as soon as possible if there is any suspicion that the encephalitis is due to herpes simplex virus. Acyclovir should be given by slow IV infusion, at a dose of 5 mg/kg over 1 hour, repeated every 8 hours. The routine use of steroid therapy in encephalitis is controversial. In mild cases it is best avoided, but in severe life-threatening viral encephalitis IV dexamethasone (adults: 4–10 mg, 6 hourly) must be given. Renal function should be rapidly assessed, and the dose of acyclovir reduced if there is evidence of renal failure. When dealing with encephalitis of uncertain cause it is usually appropriate to initiate treatment with acyclovir while awaiting the results of investigations. Expert neurological advice should be sought in all cases of severe encephalitis, especially herpes simplex encephalitis.

NON-VIRAL INFECTIVE ENCEPHALITIS

Although bacteria and other organisms commonly cause meningitis, sometimes with encephalitic features, a predominantly encephalitic picture is rare. Conditions that are associated with non-viral encephalitis include bacterial and fungal infection (particularly *Listeria monocytogenes*, Whipple's disease) and infection with Rickettsiae, spirochaetes, protozoa and Cryptococcus. Expert pathological assistance is usually required in the management of these conditions.

FURTHER READING
Johnson RT.
Viral Infections of the Nervous System. New York: Raven Press, 1987.

3. Meningitis

Acute infective meningitis may be caused by viruses, bacteria or, more rarely, other organisms. Although the clinical picture of each is sometimes distinctive, in an emergency it is foolhardy to be too categorical: many cases of clinically typical viral meningitis are subsequently identified as bacterial in origin. The signs and symptoms of meningitis can be grouped into three categories: meningeal, systemic and cerebral (Table 3.1).

VIRAL MENINGITIS

CLINICAL FEATURES
Viral meningitis is much more common than any of the other forms. The viruses that commonly cause meningitis in the UK are listed in Table 3.2; poliovirus, although rare in the UK, is an important cause of meningitis in some countries. Viral meningitis is usually mild, often occurs in

Table 3.1 Symptoms and signs of meningitis

Meningeal	Systemic	Cerebral
Headache	Fever	Encephalopathy
Stiff neck	Toxic confusion leading to delerium or even coma	Convulsions
Vomiting		
Photophobia	Specific signs*	Cranial nerve palsy
Kernig's sign		Focal signs (e.g. long-tract signs)
Bulging fontanelles in infants		

*Depending on the organism (e.g. rash in meningococcal infections, signs of tuberculosis).

Table 3.2 Causes of viral meningitis in the UK

Common	Less common
Echovirus (especially echo 9)	Adenovirus
Coxsackievirus	Lymphocytic choriomeningitis virus
Mumps virus	Herpes simplex type II
	Parainfluenza viruses
	Measles
	Epstein-Barr virus[*]

[*]Infectious mononucleosis.

epidemics, is self-limiting and has an excellent prognosis. Only systemic and meningeal signs are found; neurological signs do not normally occur.

It is often difficult initially to be certain on clinical grounds that a meningitis is viral in origin. Unless there is clear evidence of either pre-existing viral illness or definite spontaneous improvement, all cases of presumed viral meningitis should be admitted to hospital for lumbar puncture.

LABORATORY FINDINGS

The CSF typically shows a moderate lymphocytosis with a normal glucose content and negative culture (Table 3.3). The blood count may also reveal a lymphocytosis. Serial serum or CSF virological tests should show an appropriate increase in viral titres. Blood sugar should always be measured whenever a CSF sample is taken. The CSF sugar concentration is abnormal if it is less than 50% of the blood sugar concentration.

TREATMENT

No specific treatment is necessary for viral meningitis, but in severe cases fluid balance should be monitored and fever reduced. There may be viral involvement of other organs, such as the kidneys or the liver, which may require treatment. When bacterial meningitis is a diagnostic possibility, empirical antibiotic therapy should be initiated (see below and Table 3.4).

*Table 3.3 Usual findings on CSF examination in meningitis, abscess and encephalitis**

	CSF cells	Protein	Sugar	Culture
Viral meningitis	+—+++ (often lymphocytes)	↑ or →	→	Negative
Bacterial meningitis	+—+++ (usually polymorphs)	↑	↓	Positive
Tuberculous meningitis	+—+++ (usually lymphocytes)	↑	↓	Positive
Fungal meningitis	+—++ (usually lymphocytes)	↑	↓	Positive
Brain abscess	−−+	→	→	Negative
Viral encephalitis	+—++ (often lymphocytes)	↑ or →	→	Negative
Epidural/subdural abscess	+—+++ (polymorphs or lymphocytes)	↑ or →	→	Negative

*These findings are a guide only; unexpected results sometimes occur.
Cells/mm^3: −− = <5; + = 5–100; ++ = 100–500; +++ = 500–1000.
Protein and Sugar: ↑ = raised (substantially only in bacterial meningitis); → = normal; ↓ = lowered.

Table 3.4 Empirical treatment of bacterial meningitis†

Neonate	Children <6 yr	Older children and adults
Ampicillin (100 mg/kg/day) + gentamicin (2.5–7.5 mg/kg/day)	Ampicillin (400 mg/kg/day) + chloramphenicol (50–100 mg/kg/day)	benzylpenicillin (20 MU/day) + chloramphenicol (4 g/day)

†All drugs given IV in divided doses.
Penicillin may be given 2 hourly. Gentamicin and chloramphenicol dosages should be adjusted according to plasma levels.

BACTERIAL MENINGITIS

CLINICAL FEATURES

Despite the advent of antibiotics, bacterial meningitis remains a serious condition, carrying a mortality of at least 10% (up to 50% in neonates) and a considerable residual morbidity (30% in some series). The common causative organisms in the UK are listed in Table 3.5. However, other bacteria may, rarely, cause meningitis (Table 3.6), and it is imperative that accurate pathological identification is attempted in every case. Seventy-five per cent of cases occur before the age of 15 years; 15% in the first month of life. Systemic and meningeal features may occur alone or be associated with neurological signs (Table 3.1). The course and clinical picture depend upon the organism responsible, the age of the patient and any predisposing factors. The disease can be sudden and rapidly fatal, as in meningococcal meningitis, or follow a more indolent subacute course, as in tuberculous meningitis. If the presentation is acute and the progression of the disease rapid, the meningitis is almost always bacterial.

Diagnosis can be difficult, particularly in the elderly and the very young, because characteristic signs and symptoms are often absent and the meningitis may present initially with entirely non-specific symptoms. Conversely, meningism in children often occurs without meningeal

Table 3.5 Common causes of bacterial meningitis in the UK

Neonate	Children	Adults
Gram-negative bacilli*	*Haemophilus influenzae*	*Streptococcus pneumoniae*
Group B streptococci	*Streptococcus pneumoniae*	*Neisseria meningitis*
Staphylococcus aureus	*Haemophilus influenzae*	
Listeria monocytogenes		

*Especially *Escherichia coli*, *Proteus mirabilis*, *Pseudomonas aeruginosa*.

Table 3.6 Bacterial meningitis common organisms: special clinical situations

Alcoholics:	*Streptococcus pneumoniae*
	Listeria monocytogenes
CSF rhinorrhea:	*Streptococcus pneumoniae*
Endocarditis:	*Streptococcus pneumoniae*
	Staphylococcus aureus
CSF shunt:	*Staphylococcus aureus*
	Staphylococcus epidermidis
Immunosuppression:	any bacteria or other organisms

infection. The outcome depends largely on rapid diagnosis and treatment, and the most important preventable cause of permanent neurological sequelae is delay in diagnosis. Neurological sequelae are particularly common after neonatal meningitis and after pneumococcal or tuberculous meningitis in adults.

Diagnosis is based mainly on the results of CSF examination. It should be re-emphasized that, in the absence of signs of raised intracranial pressure (see below), all patients presenting with features suggestive of meningeal inflammation of unknown cause urgently require lumbar puncture.

LABORATORY FINDINGS

Table 3.7 lists the emergency investigations that should be carried out on all patients. Once meningitis is suspected, and assuming that intracranial pressure is not raised, lumbar puncture is an emergency measure. The CSF typically shows a polymorphonuclear leucocytosis and a low sugar content (Table 3.5), and organisms can be seen on microscopy and grown in culture (Table 3.3). Infecting organisms may be grown from blood cultures, even if they

Table 3.7 Emergency investigations

All cases		Selected cases	
CSF	**Blood**	**CSF**	**Other**
Cell count and differential	Bacterial culture	Microscopy using Ziehl-Nielsen or India-ink staining	Radiological
Protein	Cell count and differential		Bacterial cu
Sugar	Sugar	Culture for fungus, *Mycobacterium tuberculosis* or virus	Serological
Gram staining, microscopy and bacterial culture	Other biochemistry		
		Serological tests	
		Immunological tests	

*Depending on the clinical situation.
e.g. urea, electrolytes, liver function.
e.g. nasal, sinus, MSU.

are absent from the CSF. An obvious point, but one worth stressing, is that blood and CSF samples should be taken, whenever possible, before antibiotic treatment is initiated. The peripheral blood count usually shows a polymorphonuclear leucocytosis. Other investigations may be carried out depending on the clinical circumstances (Table 3.6).

EMERGENCY TREATMENT

Antibiotic treatment

Specific antibiotic treatment depends on the organism and should be initiated as soon as possible. Tables 3.8 and 3.9 give a guide to drugs and dosages. Expert advice should be sought for the treatment of meningitis due to unusual organisms and for patients with predisposing factors. The antibiotic sensitivities of the organisms should be determined as soon as possible and therapy adjusted accordingly.

Table 3.8 Drug therapy for specific bacterial organisms (all drugs should initially be given IV)

Organism	Treatment 1st-line	2nd-line
Neisseria meningitidis	benzylpenicillin	chloramphenicol
Streptococcus pneumoniae	benzylpenicillin	chloramphenicol
Haemophilus influenzae	chloramphenicol	ampicillin*
Gram-negative bacilli	chloramphenicol	ampicillin + gentamicin
Group B streptococci	benzylpenicillin	ampicillin
Staphylococcus aureus	flucloxacillin	gentamicin
Staphylococcus epidermidis	flucloxacillin	gentamicin
Listeria monocytogenes	ampicillin	gentamicin

*Ampicillin-resistant *Haemophilus influenzae* is increasingly common and 2nd-line therapy with cefuroxime should be considered.

Empirical antibiotic treatment should be started if identification of the organism is not immediately possible, and then changed, if necessary, when the diagnosis has been confirmed. The choice of therapy depends on the age of the patient (Table 3.4) and underlying predisposing factors. Empirical therapy should be continued until the results of cultures are available and, if they are negative, for at least three days, depending on the clinical situation.

Antibiotic treatment should be continued for at least 10 days in most cases. Penicillin should be given parenterally throughout this period, but chloramphenicol can be administered orally as soon as possible after the induction

Table 3.9 Initial IV dosages of antibiotic drugs

	Adults		Children*	
	Dose	Interval	Dose	Interval
Benzylpenicillin	20 MU/day	6×	50–100 mg/kg/day	6×
Chloramphenicol	50–100 mg/kg/day	4×	75–100 mg/kg/day	4×
Ampicillin	4–8 g/day	4×	300 mg/kg/day	4×
Gentamicin	3–5 mg/kg/day	3×	2–6 mg/kg/day	3×
Flucloxacillin	2 g/day	4×	0.5–1.0 g/day	4×
Carbenicillin	25 g/day	6×	250–400 mg/kg/day	6×
Cefuroxime	3–6 g/day	4×	100–200 mg/kg/day	4×

*excluding neonates.

of therapy. In bacterial meningitis with the common organisms, progress should be monitored on clinical grounds. Too much reliance should not be placed on repeated CSF findings, as the rate of recovery may vary considerably. Similarly, the temperature chart may also poorly reflect the patient's actual progress. In all but the most straightforward cases it is advisable to discuss the antibiotic therapy with an experienced bacteriologist, and to monitor serum levels where appropriate.

Other treatment

1. Admission to hospital is necessary for all patients, but isolation is needed only in cases of open pulmonary tuberculosis or meningococcal meningitis.

2. Fluid balance should be monitored carefully and, as most antibiotics need to be administered intravenously, a secure IV line should be set up.

3. Neurological observation at 4-hourly intervals is necessary if the patient's consciousness is impaired.

4. If seizures occur their cause should be ascertained (Table 3.10) and anticonvulsant treatment initiated immediately (Chapter 8).

5. A watch should be kept for the development of complications (Table 3.11).

Table 3.10 Causes of seizures in meningitis

Cerebral inflammation/infection
Metabolic disturbance (especially hyponatraemia)
Fever
Neurological complications
   cerebral infarction
   cerebral abscess
   subdural effusion/abscess
   cortical thrombophlebitis
   cortical vein thrombosis

Bacterial Meningitis 33

Table 3.11 Acute complications of acute bacterial meningitis

Neurological		Non-neurological
Common	**Less common**	
Cerebral infarction	Cortical vein thrombosis	DIC
Subdural effusion	Cortical thrombophlebitis	Toxaemic shock
Inappropriate ADH secretion	Obstructive hydrocephalus	Cardiorespiratory collapse
	Cerebral abscess	
Seizures	Subdural empyema	
Cerebral oedema		
Encephalopathy		
Cranial nerve palsy		

PROBLEMS IN DIAGNOSIS AND MANAGEMENT

Optic disc changes suggesting raised intracranial pressure

Intracranial pressure is raised in some cases of meningitis. This is often accompanied by slight swelling of the optic discs and, occasionally, by frank papilloedema. In cases of suspected meningitis in which the discs are only slightly engorged, lumbar puncture should be carried out and careful pressure measurements made. If the CSF is normal and the pressure high, the patient should be transferred for immediate neurological/neurosurgical investigation. If the CSF confirms a bacterial meningitis, treatment should be started immediately and a careful watch kept on the patient's neurological status. If there is any sign of deterioration, the patient should be transferred immediately for neurological/neurosurgical investigation.

If there is frank papilloedema, it is likely that the meningitis is complicated by cortical thrombophlebitis, venous sinus thrombosis, cerebral abscess or subdural empyema. Neuroradiological investigation, especially immediate CT scanning, is imperative in such cases. Lumbar puncture is contraindicated, but blood cultures should be taken. If a delay is anticipated, empirical antibiotic therapy should be initiated (p 27). A neurosurgical/neurological assessment should be organized and IV corticosteroid treatment (dexamethasone, 4–10 mg, 6-hourly) initiated while these arrangements are made.

It should also be remembered that changes of the optic disc that may be confused with papilloedema, such as haemorrhage or infiltration, may occur in a variety of conditions (e.g. hypertensive encephalopathy, blood dyscrasia, septicaemia, reticulosis, sarcoidosis).

Focal neurological signs or coma

Cerebral infarction commonly accompanies meningitis, particularly if diagnosis is delayed. Focal neurological signs (e.g. hemiparesis, cranial nerve palsy) or coma may also be caused by cerebral abscess, subdural effusion or empyema, cortical venous thrombosis or cortical thrombophlebitis. Lumbar puncture should not, therefore, be carried out until after urgent neuroradiological and neurological/neurosurgical assessment.

Partially treated meningitis

If a patient with bacterial meningitis is given inappropriate antibiotic treatment before the causative organism has been identified, the CSF tends to normalize, although it seldom becomes completely normal. There may be cells but no organisms, and culture will be sterile. This may pose a considerable diagnostic problem for the emergency physician, and there is a serious risk of relapse or chronic meningitis. It is an avoidable situation that is, unfortunately, all too common. *Ideally no case of bacterial meningitis should receive antibiotics until blood and CSF specimens have been obtained for culture* (except if meningococcal meningitis is suspected).

In such partially treated cases, empirical treatment should be started (Table 3.4) and repeated lumbar punctures and blood cultures carried out. Progress may be monitored by changes in the CSF white cell count and in the patient's neurological status.

Sterile meningitis

If a patient shows a clinical picture of meningitis and characteristic CSF changes (e.g. cells, protein, sugar) but no organism is seen or cultured by conventional methods, this is known as a 'sterile meningitis'. The common causes of this condition are listed in Table 3.12. The history may give

Table 3.12 Common causes of sterile meningitis

Partially treated bacterial meningitis
Tuberculous meningitis
Viral meningitis
Fungal meningitis
Cerebral abscess
Subdural abscess/empyema
Cortical thrombophlebitis
Carcinomatous meningitis
Sarcoidosis
Meningovascular syphilis

clues to the aetiology. A rash or pleurodynia, for instance, suggest enterovirus infection; or a history of travel or occupational exposure, poliomyelitis or leptospirosis. In cases of partially treated bacterial meningitis, the cells are often polymorphonuclear and the CSF glucose level is usually low. In a viral infection the CSF cells are often mononuclear and the glucose content is usually normal. The tubercle bacillus is notoriously difficult to see using light microscopy and takes many weeks to grow in culture, hence tuberculous meningitis may often present as a sterile meningitis. In tuberculous meningitis the CSF glucose level is usually very low, the protein content often very high and there may be other evidence of tuberculosis. The CSF should be examined meticulously on several occasions for acid-fast bacilli. Fungal meningitis is rare in this country unless the patient is immunosuppressed, and the organisms may be detected by India-ink staining of concentrated CSF. Cases of carcinomatous meningitis may present with a low CSF sugar content, suggesting infection, but cytological examination of concentrated CSF will usually show malignant cells.

In most emergencies, empirical therapy should be given (Table 3.4). If the clinical and CSF findings are suggestive of tuberculous infection and the neurological status of the patient is deteriorating, anti-tuberculous therapy may also be started while awaiting the results of culture.

Recurrent meningitis

Recurrent meningitis poses another difficult clinical

problem, particularly as the causative organisms may be atypical. The usual predisposing factors are an anatomical defect resulting in a breach in the meningeal covering (e.g. meningomyelocoele, skull fracture), a chronic parameningeal infection (e.g. sinusitis, mastoiditis, osteomyelitis) or impaired immunity. Depending on the likely cause, it may be necessary to look at the results of nasal or skin cultures prior to starting treatment.

Neonatal meningitis

Meningitis is relatively common in the neonate (1/2500 live births), and is a serious condition with a high mortality and morbidity. A wide range of pathogens may be responsible, making treatment difficult. The commonest causative organisms in the UK are *Escherichia coli*, the beta-haemolytic streptococci, *Listeria monocytogenes, Proteus mirabilis, Pseudomonas aeruginosa* and *Staphylococcus aureus*.

Diagnosis can be difficult as conventional signs of meningitis may be entirely absent and other symptoms (e.g. respiratory distress) may suggest other conditions. Lumbar puncture and blood culture should be carried out at the earliest possible opportunity. Parenteral ampicillin and gentamicin are the most commonly used antibiotics; chloramphenicol, carbenicillin, amikacin and kanamycin can also be used, depending on the sensitivities of the isolated organisms. Achieving *appropriate* antibiotic concentrations in the meningeal space can be a problem. Although some authorities recommend intrathecal administration of some antibiotics (e.g. aminoglycosides), this route is best avoided except in specialized units. Chloramphenicol is particularly toxic in the newborn and may cause the 'grey baby syndrome'.

Commonly, too high a dose of chloramphenicol is given. The usual recommendation for pre-term neonates and neonates in the first week of life is a dose of 25 mg/kg/day, and for neonates >7 days old a dose of 37.5–50 mg/kg/day. Where ever possible, repeated serum levels should be obtained and the dosage thereafter tailored to the results. In neonates, in contrast to children and adults, because absorption is unreliable, oral administration is not

Tuberculous meningitis

This condition is seen increasingly often in hospital practice; it may be difficult to diagnose and the outcome depends largely on the speed with which diagnosis is made and treatment initiated. It usually presents in a subacute form with early non-specific symptoms (e.g. malaise, lethargy, indolent fever). Progressive meningeal and neurological symptoms then appear, including headache, stiff neck, seizures, mental changes, cranial nerve palsies and long-tract signs.

Diagnosis is sometimes facilitated by an abnormal chest X-ray or elevated ESR, but a definite diagnosis depends on the isolation and culture of tuberculous organisms from the CSF. These may be hard to detect and slow to culture, and it is often necessary to repeat the CSF examinations. CSF protein is often very high and CSF sugar very low. The CSF cell-type is predominantly lymphocytic in established cases, but only polymorphs may be present initially (Table 3.3). Unfortunately, these changes are neither consistent nor diagnostic. Triple therapy should be initiated as soon as possible and is advisable in a patient whose clinical picture is suggestive, even if CSF microscopy is negative. Specific anti-tuberculous therapy may have to wait for several weeks before the sensitivities of the organisms can be ascertained. Acute complications (e.g. cranial nerve palsy, encephalopathy, cerebral infarction) are frequent. As these complications are due to arteritis, some authorities recommend the regular use of steroid therapy in the acute stage, but there is no conclusive evidence that this is helpful.

OTHER FORMS OF INFECTIVE MENINGITIS

FUNGAL MENINGITIS

This is most frequently found in patients with immunological disorders, debilitating diseases, haematological disorders, chronic renal disease, AIDS or immunosuppressive therapy. The commonest causative organisms in the UK are *Cryptococcus neoformans* (torulosis) and Candida. The course of the meningitis is usually chronic and the outcome often poor. Diagnosis can be difficult. CSF examination usually shows a lymphocytic leucocytosis, high protein and reduced glucose. The organisms are often difficult to detect without special staining, difficult to culture and, indeed, often absent from the specimen; hence, repeated CSF examinations may be necessary. Both cryptococcal and candidal meningitis are treated initially with amphotericin B (0.3 mg/kg/day as a slow IV infusion) and oral flucytosine (150 mg/kg/day) in four divided doses. However, the fungus may persist despite treatment, and expert advice is essential in the management of such cases.

MENINGOVASCULAR SYPHILIS

Neurosyphilis may present as acute or subacute meningitis (meningovascular syphilis). The diagnosis can be rapidly established by serological testing of the CSF. This should be carried out in all cases of 'sterile meningitis'. Treatment is with procaine penicillin (1 MU IM daily for 21 days), covered initially by oral prednisone (40 mg daily for 3 days) to prevent a Herxheimer reaction.

OTHER

Other forms of infective meningitis (e.g. parasitic meningitis) are exceedingly rare in the UK and present as a sterile meningitis, usually with specific systemic signs. It is important to emphasize that all cases of sterile meningitis need urgent investigation as the course is often progressive and the causes are serious.

FURTHER READING

Lambert HP.
Meningitis. In: Harrison MJG, ed. *Contemporary Neurology*. Butterworths: London, 1984; 314–21.

4. Intracranial Abscess and Venous Thrombosis/ Thrombophlebitis

Localized infection may occur in brain tissue (cerebral abscess), the subdural space (subdural empyema) or the extradural space (extradural abscess). These infections are much less common than meningitis, but they are potentially serious and require urgent identification and treatment. Non-infective or infective thrombosis of the cerebral veins or sinuses can also occur, often following or complicating intracranial abscess or meningitis. These conditions may all present as neurological emergencies and are dealt with together in this chapter.

CEREBRAL ABSCESS

In a patient with normal immune responses, cerebral abscess is usually bacterial. There are three principal causes.
1. Spreading infection from middle ear or sinus sepsis — infection may extend from the ear or mastoid to the adjacent temporal lobes, or from the nasal sinuses to the frontal lobe.
2. Open head injury or surgery.
3. Haematogenous spread from a site of systemic infection, particularly a pulmonary abscess or endocarditis, but any primary source of infection may metastasize. Patients with cyanotic congenital heart disease or congenital pulmonary angiomatous lesions seem especially susceptible.

The type of organism responsible depends on the source of the infection, and many different pathogens have been reported; the most common in the UK are anaerobic bacteria (in contrast to meningitis), *Staphylococcus aureus*,

Streptococcus pneumoniae, Haemophilus influenzae, other streptococci, Gram-negative cocci and *Mycobacterium tuberculosis*. Sometimes, more than one organism is responsible and, occasionally, a non-bacterial fungal or parasitic abscess may occur.

Cerebral abscess is also increasingly common in immunocompromised patients (e.g. those on immunosuppressive drugs, those with malignant diseases, haematological diseases, AIDS or other immunological disorders). In such cases the organisms may be unusual and the course of the abscess atypical. Diagnosis can be very difficult. Cerebral abscess has a poor prognosis, with 30%–70% mortality and high neurological morbidity. Early diagnosis and treatment are essential to minimize these risks.

CLINICAL FEATURES

Bacterial cerebral abscess usually has a subacute course, and the early stages are notoriously difficult to diagnose (Table 4.1). Early symptoms may be non-specific (e.g. malaise, fever and loss of appetite). Specific neurological symptoms will then appear, by which time action is urgently needed. These include symptoms of raised intracranial pressure, which may be prominent, alterations of behaviour or consciousness, seizures, the development of focal neurological symptoms and meningism. In some cases the history may be very acute. Signs may include fever, meningism, confusion, depressed consciousness, focal neurological deficit and papilloedema. *The presence of focal*

Table 4.1 Clinical features of cerebral abscess.

Non-specific, particularly in the early stages
Infection (e.g. fever, toxaemia)
Raised intracranial pressure (e.g. headache, altered mental state, depression of consciousness, papilloedema)
Seizures
Focal neurological signs (e.g. aphasia, hemiparesis, cranial nerve palsy)
Meningism

neurological signs, seizures or raised intracranial pressure (e.g. papilloedema) in a patient with fever or signs of infection is a strong indication of cerebral abscess.

INVESTIGATIONS

CT

The principal emergency investigation is the CT scan. This should be arranged immediately in all cases of suspected abscess, even if out of hours. At a very early stage of 'cerebritis' — before an abscess has developed — the scan may be normal; later, however, it is always abnormal and usually diagnostic (Fig 4.1).

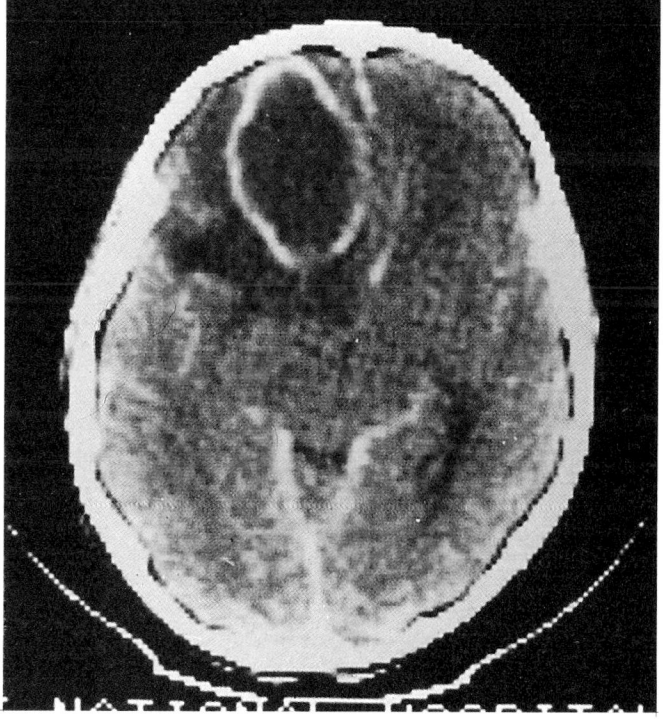

Figure 4.1 CT Showing cerebral abscess. Kindly donated by Dr G. Tatler.

Lumbar puncture
Lumbar puncture is contraindicated in cases of suspected abscess, as the risk of transtentorial coning is considerable (see p 14). The temptation to obtain CSF from a patient with fever/meningism, focal neurological signs and/or signs of raised intracranial pressure should be resisted.

Cerebral angiography/EEG
Cerebral angiography should be performed if CT scanning is not available, but prior to this a specialist neurological or neurosurgical opinion should be sought. The EEG may be helpful but is seldom diagnostic, and the time taken to organize this would be better spent arranging for a CT scan or transfer to a neurological unit.

Culture/haematology/biochemistry
Blood culture, a complete blood count and biochemical analysis of serum should be carried out as an emergency procedure.

Other
The primary source of infection should be sought; this may involve further radiological or bacteriological investigations.

EMERGENCY TREATMENT
In almost all cases the primary treatment of cerebral abscess is neurosurgical excision or aspiration; therefore, all cases of proven abscess should be transferred immediately to a neurosurgical or neurological unit. Occasionally, surgery may not be the best initial option, but this will require specialist consideration and the patient is best treated in a neurological setting. While neurosurgical transfer is being arranged, an IV line should be set up and IV steroid therapy instituted (dexamethasone, 4–10 mg, 6-hourly). Prophylactic anticonvulsant therapy with phenytoin should also be started (Chapter 8). If signs of transtentorial herniation (coning) develop, emergency treatment may be required (see p 14).

At operation, a bacteriological sample should be sent for microscopy and culture; further treatment will depend on the results. In exceptional cases broad-spectrum antibiotic therapy should be started if neurosurgical intervention is to be delayed; however, this may render subsequent bacteriological identification impossible and seriously compromise further management. The choice of antibiotics depends on the clinical situation and the cultured organism, but will usually include penicillin, chloramphenicol, metronidazole, trimethoprim and sulphamethoxazole.

INTRACRANIAL SUBDURAL EMPYEMA

This is usually a complication of frontal sinusitis, but also occurs occasionally in sphenoidal sinusitis and ear disease. The subdural space is potentially large and the empyema may develop rapidly and spread over a large area. The empyema can cause raised intracranial pressure; in addition, secondary cortical inflammatory changes, arteritis and cerebral venous thrombosis/thrombophlebitis may occur, causing focal neurological signs.

CLINICAL FEATURES

The clinical features are: signs of infection, including fever and/or toxaemia (these are invariable and can be severe); seizures; alterations in the mental state or level of consciousness and signs of raised intracranial pressure; and focal neurological signs (e.g. aphasia, hemiplegia). The clinical course may be rapid and fulminating and the mortality and risk of residual neurological disability are high; these can be minimized only by early diagnosis and treatment.

DIAGNOSIS

CT scanning may be helpful, but if the abscess is small it may be obscured by artifacts from the skull bones. Cerebral angiography is diagnostic, and a neurosurgical opinion should be sought. Usually, transfer to a neurosurgical unit should be arranged as rapidly as possible. CSF examination is contraindicated as intracranial pressure may be raised, but blood cultures and cultures from the site of infection should

INTRACRANIAL ABSCESS

be obtained.

EMERGENCY TREATMENT
The principles of treatment are similar to those for cerebral abscess. Urgent neurosurgical intervention is required and the abscess should be drained and appropriate antibiotic treatment initiated.

INTRACRANIAL EXTRADURAL ABSCESS

Intracranial extradural abscesses usually form after sinus or ear infection. The abscess is outside the dura, usually small and does not cause raised intracranial pressure. Focal signs and convulsions are less common although a spreading arteritis, which can affect the cerebral cortex, may occur. The predominant signs are therefore those of infection and focal neurological deficit. The principles of diagnosis and

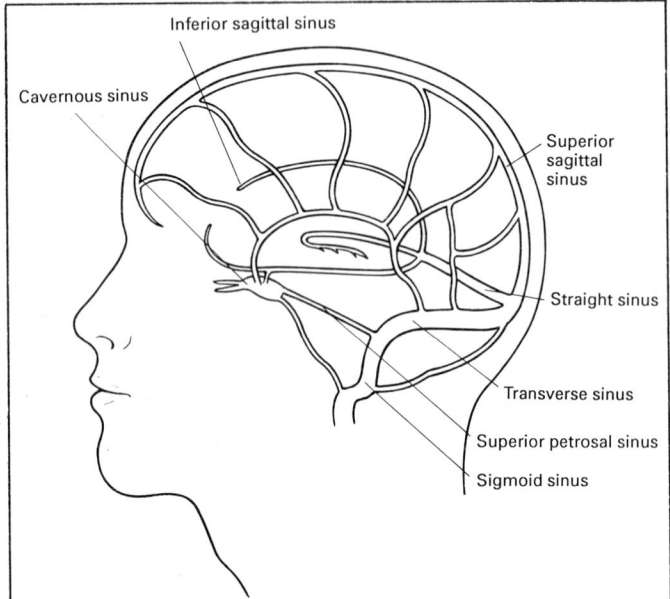

Figure 4.2 The large cerebral veins and venous sinuses.

treatment are similar to those for a cerebral abscess and a subdural empyema. Radiological studies may be diagnostic, the CSF usually shows a pleocytosis, and treatment consists of antibiotics and surgical drainage.

CEREBRAL VENOUS THROMBOSIS/ THROMBOPHLEBITIS

These are probably more frequent than is generally recognised and the diagnosis, particularly of a non-infective cortical venous thrombosis, is often missed. Two types of venous thrombosis/thrombophlebitis may present as a neurological emergency. The severity of the thrombus depends on the sinus or vein involved (Fig 4.2) and the extent of the circulatory disturbance.

CORTICAL VEIN THROMBOSIS/ THROMBOPHLEBITIS

These may occur in isolation or be accompanied by dural sinus thrombosis. The thrombosis may cause haemorrhage into the subarachnoid space and the brain.

The clinical features are those of infection (where present), cerebral cortical disturbance and, sometimes, raised intracranial pressure. They include severe headache (usually a predominant feature), fever, toxaemia, nausea, vomiting, neck stiffness, seizures (sometimes status epilepticus), impaired consciousness (sometimes coma), focal neurological signs (e.g. aphasia, hemiparesis) and papilloedema.

In some cases the clinical course is sudden and rapidly progressive and often the patients are gravely ill, whereas in other cases the course is subacute or insidious. These conditions are particularly common in childhood where they may occur subsequent to dehydration, fever or infection. Young children in particular may present subacutely, with failure to thrive, weight loss, etc. In adults there are a number of common predisposing factors (Table 4.2) but often no cause is found.

Table 4.2 Predisposing causes for cortical vein thrombosis in adults

Infection (especially sinus, mastoid, ear, meningitis, intracranial abscess)
Dehydration, fever or metabolic disorders
Altered coagulation states (e.g. pregnancy, puerperium or contraceptive pill)
Systemic disorders (e.g. malignancy, diabetes, Behcet's syndrome or Budd-Chiari syndrome)
Haematological disorders (e.g. leukaemia, polycythaemia, haemolytic anaemia, thrombocytopenia)
Head trauma or intracranial surgery

CAVERNOUS SINUS THROMBOSIS/ THROMBOPHLEBITIS

These usually follow infection of the nasal sinuses, ocular or facial tissues and, as there is free communication between the sinuses, are generally bilateral.

The clinical features are those of systemic symptoms of infection, focal signs of venous engorgement of the cavernous sinus and the ophthalmic and retinal veins, and involvement of related structures such as the optic and oculomotor nerves. The signs and symptoms are fever, toxaemia, headache, ocular pain, tenderness, proptosis, chemosis, periorbital oedema, paresis of cranial nerves III, IV, VI and the ophthalmic division of V (causing ptosis and ocular palsy), papilloedema and, sometimes, blurring of vision. These patients are usually gravely ill.

DIAGNOSIS

This is based essentially on clinical findings and, although usually straightforward in cavernous sinus thrombosis, may be much more difficult in cortical vein thrombosis. A high index of clinical suspicion is needed and the diagnosis should be considered in any person presenting with severe headache, seizures, a deteriorating level of consciousness, increasing toxaemia or focal neurological signs, particularly in the presence of a focal infection.

INVESTIGATIONS

In the emergency room, blood should be sent off for a full

blood count, ESR and culture, and swabs taken of any possible infection site. Arrangements should be made for transfer to a neurological/neurosurgical unit and CT organized. This may be normal or show oedema or patchy haemorrhagic infarction. CT will also help to exclude other structural intracranial lesions. Lumbar puncture may be necessary to exclude meningitis and may show evidence of haemorrhage or simply raised protein levels and a moderate pleocytosis. The pressure will be elevated, sometimes markedly, and lumbar puncture carries some risk. Cerebral angiography is usually diagnostic, but this must be carried out in an experienced unit.

EMERGENCY TREATMENT

Establish/treat underlying cause
The underlying cause (e.g. infection or dehydration) should be established and treated. If infection is present, as is commonly the case, this should be treated immediately with appropriate antibiotics (Chapter 3).

Seizures
Seizures should be controlled (Chapter 8).

Other
In the majority of cases no active treatment of the thrombosis is indicated. Although anticoagulants have been advocated by some, haemorrhagic infarction is often also present and the use of these drugs is hazardous. IV dexamethasone (4–10 mg, 6-hourly) is often given, but there is no clear evidence that this is helpful.

5. Stroke and Subarachnoid Haemorrhage

STROKE

Although stroke is the commonest neurological emergency, it is often poorly managed in its acute stages. In the elderly, emergency admission to hospital may be inappropriate, but if the patient is kept at home it is essential to monitor progress carefully. Admission to hospital is advisable, however, for all patients under 50, all patients when there is doubt about the diagnosis, all patients with a treatable underlying cause, and the elderly patient who will not receive adequate supportive care at home. Once admitted, the extent of investigation and the vigor of intensive early treatment depend on the age of the patient, the underlying cause of the stroke and other clinical and domestic factors. Such decisions may be difficult in the emergency setting, and a careful medical and social history from relatives or the patient's general practitioner is essential.

DIAGNOSIS

A stroke is usually easy to diagnose. It is characterized by the sudden onset of a neurological disturbance, with a subsequent tendency to recovery, sometimes with altered consciousness, headache or vomiting. The exact neurological symptoms depend on the site of the damage. Diagnosis may be difficult if the presentation is atypical, an adequate history is unavailable or, particularly, the patient is confused or unconscious. Furthermore, not all acute neurological episodes are due to stroke, and to make this assumption is to court disaster. The conditions most commonly mistaken for stroke are listed in Table 5.1. Many of these can be excluded by clinical examination or by simple investigation

50 Stroke and Subarachnoid Haemorrhage

Table 5.1 Conditions commonly misdiagnosed as stroke

Intracranial tumour (primary and secondary)
Subdural haematoma
Extradural haematoma
Cerebral abscess
Encephalitis
Epileptic seizure
Multiple sclerosis (acute relapse)
Hysterical conversion
Other causes of coma (Chapter 1)
Other causes of transient cerebral ischaemia (e.g. cardiac arrhythmia, hypoglycaemia, migraine)

in the emergency room. In the diagnosis of stroke, attention should be directed towards the differentiation between haemorrhage and infarction, and the identification of the site of cerebral damage and the underlying cause.

Differentiation between haemorrhage and infarction

This is important, but cannot be made clinically. Compared with infarction, haemorrhage is more often associated with a sudden onset, headache, vomiting, alteration of

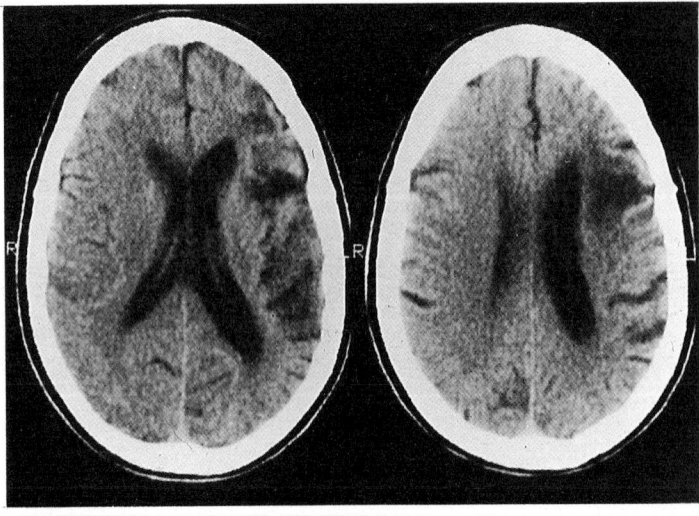

Figure 5.1 CT scans showing cerebral infarction. Kindly donated by Dr G. Tatler.

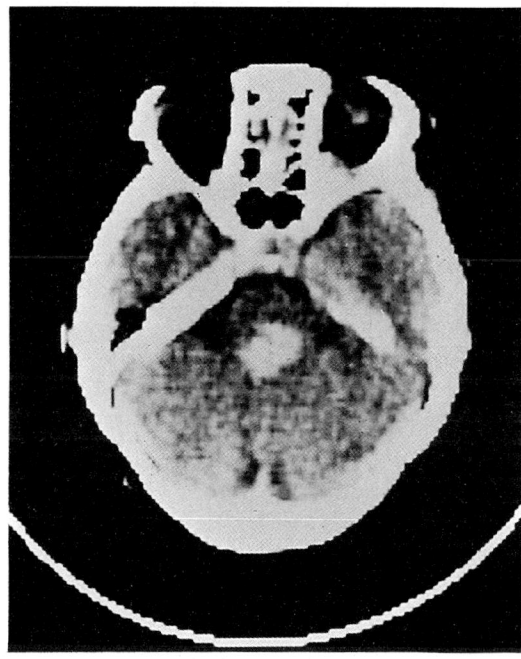

Figure 5.2 CT scan showing intracerebral haemorrhage. Kindly donated by Dr G. Tatler

consciousness and hypertension. However, these differences are not absolute and of little diagnostic assistance in the individual patient. CT is the only reliable routine non-invasive method of making this distinction (Figs. 5.1 and 5.2). Lumbar puncture may help but it should be remembered that if the haemorrhage is confined to intracerebral tissue the CSF may not contain blood.

Identification of the site of damage

This is often possible clinically, although with the advent of CT it has become clear that clinical localization is frequently inaccurate. In cerebral infarction distinction should be made between carotid and vertebrobasilar territory involvement and, if possible, involvement of specific cerebral arteries (Table 5.2) as further management and prognosis depend on the site and extent of cerebral damage. In all cases stroke

Table 5.2 Clinical features of stroke in specific cerebral artery territories.

Anterior and middle cerebral arteries, internal carotid artery	Posterior cerebral artery	Vertebral artery
Hemiparesis*	Hemianopia	Pupillary abnormalities
Hemisensory loss*	Visual, visiospatial agnosia	Eye movement disorders
Hemianopia		
Dysphasia (if dominant)	Seizures (uncommon)	Cranial nerve signs
Personality, behavioural changes		Dysarthria
		Dysphagia
Dyspraxia, agnosia, other psychological changes		Unilateral/bilateral motor/sensory loss
		Cerebellar signs
Incontinence		Tremor, extrapyramidal signs
Seizures		
		Hemianopia
		Visual, visiospatial agnosia

*Anterior cerebral artery - leg affected more than arm. Middle cerebral artery - arm and face affected more than leg.

may be associated with headache, alterations of consciousness, drowsiness and vomiting. Occlusion of the internal carotid usually produces symptoms of middle cerebral artery damage, but the exact sequelae depend on the adequacy of cross-flow in the circle of Willis.

Identification of the underlying cause
Most strokes are the result of degenerative arterial disease, but in a minority of cases — particularly in the younger patient — there are other causative factors (Table 5.3).

These may require urgent treatment.

Table 5.3 Medical conditions causing stroke

Degenerative arterial disease
Hypertensive vascular disease
Cardiac disease
   arrhythmia (of any kind, especially atrial fibrillation)
   myocardial infarction
   valvular disease (rheumatic, congenital, ischaemic)
   endocarditis (of any kind)
   cardiomyopathy
   atrial myxoma
Haematological disease
   leukaemia and reticulosis
   polycythaemia
   other, rarer causes (e.g. sickle cell disease)
Clotting and coagulation defects
Trauma to head or neck
Infection
   bacterial endocarditis
   septicaemia, meningitis, cerebral abscess and other intracranial infection
   neurosyphilis
   infection spreading to extracranial carotid artery (e.g. tonsilitis)
Vasculitis
   collagen diseases (e.g. SLE)
   giant cell arteritis
   other rarer arteritides (e.g. Takayasu arteritis, granulomatous angiitis, sarcoid angiitis, syphilitic angiitis)
Carotid artery disease
   atheroma/occulsion
   other, rarer causes (e.g. dissection, fibromuscular dysplasia)
Miscellaneous
   structural intracranial lesions (e.g. angioma)
   contraceptive pill
   hyperviscosity syndromes (e.g. in myeloma, other hyperproteinaemia, cryoglobulinaemia)
   blood lipid disorders

EMERGENCY INVESTIGATIONS

General investigations

Measurements of serum levels of urea, glucose and electrolytes, a full blood count and ESR should be made in all patients. An ECG should be performed if there is any suspicion of cardiac disease (a silent myocardial infarction may present as stroke). A chest X-ray may also be helpful in identifying cardiac or pulmonary disease. Other urgent investigations depend on the clinical circumstances and include blood culture, protein electrophoresis, plasma lipids, antinuclear factor, DNA binding, sickle cell screen, temporal artery biopsy, syphilitic serology, echocardiogram.

CT and skull X-ray

CT will allow definitive diagnosis and localization of intracerebral haemorrhage, subdural or extradural haemorrhage, and most cases of infarction. It will also help to differentiate stroke from other structural cerebral disorders. Although its use in acute stroke depends on local facilities and the clinical situation, CT will minimize diagnostic error and identify treatable pathology. If CT is unavailable, a skull X-ray may identify shift of the intracranial mid-line structures or abnormal calcification, but it is otherwise of little help in acute stroke; an isotope scan is likewise of limited usefulness.

Cerebral angiography

Angiography is only very occasionally required in the acute stage of stroke. It is associated with an appreciable morbidity, and the decision to proceed to angiography should be made in consultation with a neurologist or neurosurgeon. The indications for its use depend on local facilities and on the circumstances of the individual patient, but are broadly confined to (i) the young patient, within a few hours of the onset of the stroke, in whom acute carotid thrombosis is suspected and carotid endarterectomy is planned; (ii) the young patient with a traumatic carotid occlusion (e.g. in a road-traffic accident or fall); and (iii) patients with possible cerebral haemorrhage whose neurological condition is deteriorating and for whom surgical removal of the haemorrhage is contemplated. All are rare indications.

Lumbar puncture

Lumbar puncture is potentially dangerous if intracranial pressure is raised and should be carried out in selected patients only. Its most common indications are to assist in the diagnosis of subarachnoid haemorrhage, and to exclude meningitis, encephalitis or, as a prelude to anticoagulation. If a lumbar puncture is to be carried out, it is advisable to perform CT beforehand to exclude an intracranial mass. CT itself will often provide the relevant diagnostic information.

EMERGENCY MANAGEMENT

Although numerous therapies have been recommended to limit the initial damage in acute stroke, in practice none have been shown conclusively to improve morbidity. There is little or no place for steroids, osmotic agents, vasodilators, dextran, inhaled carbon dioxide or hyperventilation; indeed they may worsen the outcome. In certain situations, however, further active treatment is warranted.

Anticoagulants

Opinions vary about the value of these drugs. In acute stroke the only definite indications are in small infarcts due to embolism associated with atrial fibrillation in the presence of mitral stenosis or an artificial heart valve. Their usefulness in other situations is doubtful. Whenever anticoagulants are to be used, prior CT and lumbar puncture should be carried out to exclude haemorrhage. Anticoagulation should be initiated with heparin and maintained with warfarin.

Antihypertensive agents

Blood pressure rises in the first few days after stroke in many cases, hence a high blood pressure on admission does not necessarily mean that the patient has chronic hypertension. If blood pressure is lowered too quickly in the acute phase of stroke, further cerebral damage may occur; therefore, no immediate antihypertensive treatment should be instituted unless the blood pressure is very high (diastolic >120 mmHg or systolic >220 mmHg, depending on age). If hypertension persists >48 hours, however, it should be treated along normal clinical lines.

Emergency surgery

The vogue for immediate angiography and carotid endarterectomy in a 'stroke in evolution' or in acute carotid thrombosis has passed, and now only a few centres recommend this approach. It is reserved for the young stroke patient who can be examined within an hour or two of onset or who has a traumatic carotid thrombosis. Surgical evacuation of an intracranial haematoma is likewise seldom of benefit and should be considered only in patients with a large haemorrhage whose neurological status is progressively deteriorating or in some patients with a cerebellar haematoma.

General measures

These are very important in all stroke patients. Hydration should be maintained but over-hydration avoided as it may increase cerebral damage, and serum electrolytes and glucose levels monitored. If there is paralysis, the patient should be nursed carefully; undue stretching or secondary injury to the paralysed limbs should be avoided and skin and eye care and passive movements initiated. The airway must be protected and hypoxia, which may worsen cerebral ischaemia, avoided or corrected. Seizures should be treated immediately (Chapter 8). Constipation should be avoided. Haemoconcentration may worsen cerebral ischaemia; if the haematocrit is >0.45, venesection should be considered. Hypotension carries a poor prognosis and should be corrected. Aspiration pneumonia, urinary tract infection, deep vein thrombosis, pulmonary embolism, leg ulceration, contracture and frozen shoulder are avoidable complications. Finally, and most importantly, the patient and family should be treated with sensitivity and attentiveness.

SUBARACHNOID HAEMORRHAGE

DIAGNOSIS

Subarachnoid haemorrhage is a common and important neurological emergency. Causes include a ruptured cerebral aneurysm or, more rarely, an arteriovenous malformation, haematological or clotting disorder or mycotic aneurysm. In a few patients no cause can be detected.

The diagnosis can usually be made in the emergency room. The history is often characteristic, with a sudden onset of severe headache, vomiting, photophobia and neck stiffness. Consciousness may be lost. Examination will show nuchal rigidity, a positive Kernig's sign and variable degrees of drowsiness and focal neurological signs, depending on associated cerebral damage. A subhyaloid retinal haemorrhage is occasionally found and this is very helpful in confirming the diagnosis. All patients should be admitted to hospital in the acute phase.

EMERGENCY INVESTIGATIONS

CT often reveals blood in the subarachnoid space or ventricles, and this is the investigation of choice. Lumbar puncture may confer some risk for patients with large haemorrhages or critically raised intracranial pressure; therefore it should not be carried out routinely but reserved for cases in which the CT is normal or, if CT is not available, for suspected cases with preserved consciousness and no marked focal signs. In other situations, it may be best to seek advice from the neurologist or neurosurgeon regarding further investigation. If lumbar puncture is withheld there is a danger of missing a case of meningitis or of failing to make a positive diagnosis, complicating future management. An emergency full blood count, ESR, measurements of blood urea, glucose and electrolytes, and a clotting profile should be obtained in all patients.

EMERGENCY MANAGEMENT

General measures
These are similar to those in stroke (see p 56).

Prevention of further haemorrhage
The aim of further management in subarachnoid haemorrhage due to an intracranial aneurysm is to prevent a re-bleed, which is a substantial risk within the first few weeks. General management includes strict bed rest, preferably in quiet surroundings, measures taken to avoid stress, laxative medication and, in some cases, mild sedation. Blood pressure should be carefully monitored and hypertension cautiously treated from the onset. Antifibrinolytic drugs probably have no part to play in the routine management of subarachnoid haemorrhage.

Early angiography and surgery should be considered in two situations. First, in all patients <65 years who are alert and have no prominent neurological signs. Early surgery may substantially reduce the long-term morbidity. Transfer to a neurosurgical unit should be arranged, ideally within 48 hours of the bleed. Four-vessel angiography is usually undertaken in those <50 years, and carotid angiography is usually performed in those aged 50–65. The timing of angiography depends on local neurosurgical practice. Early angiography and surgery should not be undertaken in patients >65 or in any patient with severe impairment of consciousness or marked focal signs; such patients should be managed medically, at least initially.

Second, it should be considered in patients with an intracerebral haematoma, particularly those with a cerebellar haematoma, whose neurological status is deteriorating. Surgical evacuation of the haematoma may help in some cases although the outlook is generally poor. Expert neurosurgical advice should be sought. Some patients deteriorate within the first week of the bleed owing to spasm of intracerebral arteries, which may be difficult to distinguish from a second haemorrhage. If deterioration occurs in a patient being managed medically, urgent neurological advice should be obtained. The mechanism of arterial spasm is unclear. Calcium channel blockers (eg Nimodipine) have recently proved useful in preventing spasm, but there are no other reliable methods of either predicting or treating it.

FURTHER READING

Ross Russell R, ed.
Vascular Diseases of the Central Nervous System. 2nd ed.
Edinburgh: Churchill Livingstone, 1984.

6. Head Injury

Trauma to the head is very common. In the UK over 100 000 patients are admitted to hospital each year with a head injury; an even greater number attend a casualty department and are then discharged. Most cases are mild and require no specific treatment, but a small number are seriously injured and the identification and correct early management of these patients, who are often at risk of severe neurological damage, is vital.

Cerebral damage following head trauma can be caused in various ways: acceleration and deceleration forces may result in widespread small contusions and lacerations; less commonly, a larger vessel is torn causing a localized intracerebral, subdural or extradural haemorrhage. Localized cerebral damage may be caused by a depressed skull fracture. Localized or generalized brain swelling may cause raised intracranial pressure. Secondary hydrocephalus may result from damage to the CSF circulation or from bleeding into the ventricles. Finally, extracranial injury may result in secondary brain damage, such as that caused by anoxia, hypotension or systemic emboli.

INITIAL ASSESSMENT

A detailed history should be taken and an examination carried out, the findings of which should be recorded scrupulously; this is important both for subsequent assessment and for medico-legal reasons. Other injuries, if present, should also be evaluated carefully. Serious orthopaedic or abdominal injuries may be easily overlooked in the comatose patient; conversely, in the conscious patient with multiple injuries, significant head trauma may be neglected. However priorities must be established — a

Table 6.1 Criteria for performing skull X-ray after recent head injury*

Loss of consciousness
Amnesia
Neurological symptoms or signs
CSF or blood from nose or ear
Suspected penetrating injury
Scalp bruising or swelling
Difficulty in assessing the patient (e.g. with epilepsy, alcohol intoxication, children)

*The above are guidelines only; use clinical judgement. (Adopted from guidelines of the Department of Neurosurgery, Institute of Neurological Sciences, Glasgow, UK.)

developing cerebral haematoma takes precedence over a compound limb fracture.

The patient should be assessed for respiratory insufficiency or shock, and blood gases may need to be measured. If the airway is obstructed or threatened, or ventilation is inadequate, the patient should be intubated and ventilated immediately.

It is important to detect skull fracture, hence a skull X-ray should be carried out (Table 6.1), and repeated if it is of inadequate quality. Fractures are not usually associated with overt clinical signs, although occasionally a fracture line may be seen in a scalp laceration. Other clinical clues to the presence of a fracture include bleeding or CSF leakage from the nose or ear in basal fractures, postauricular bruising in fractures of the petrous bone and orbital bruising in fractures of the anterior fossa. Special views of a suspicious area should be taken and the X-ray results reported immediately.

In the casualty department scalp lacerations should be carefully examined, cleaned and sutured, and mild headache treated with a simple analgesic. If admission to hospital is not justified, the patient or responsible adult should be given written instructions explaining the need to return to the casualty department should neurological symptoms develop.

ADMISSION TO HOSPITAL

The patient who is comatose or otherwise severely injured should of course be admitted (Table 6.2). All patients with a skull fracture or a suspected skull fracture should likewise be admitted to hospital. However, admission may also be necessary for less severe cases depending on a number of factors, including post-traumatic amnesia — the period from the accident to the time when the patient is able to recall ongoing events. It is longer than the period of 'unconsciousness' as judged by witnesses. The degree of generalized cerebral dysfunction may be accurately assessed by the duration of the post-traumatic amnesia and it is wise to admit all patients with post-traumatic amnesia of more than a few minutes. All patients with severe headache, confusion or impairment of consciousness should be admitted, as should those who have experienced focal neurological symptoms/signs or seizures.

Many patients with head trauma have taken alcohol, which may complicate the neurological assessment. Nevertheless, it is foolhardy to attribute any drowsiness or change in behaviour to alcohol without good evidence, and it is safer to admit all patients when there is any doubt. A blood alcohol measurement may be very useful in this situation. Similarly, patients with complicating medical conditions (e.g. on anticoagulants) should also be admitted, as should those who cannot be properly supervised at home.

Table 6.2 Criteria for admission to hospital

Coma
Other severe injury
Skull fracture
Post-traumatic amnesia (most cases)
Headache (most cases)
Confusion
Impairment of consciousness
Focal neurological symptoms/signs
Seizures
Complicating medical conditions
Lack of supervision out of hospital

EARLY HOSPITAL MANAGEMENT

THE UNCONSCIOUS PATIENT

The early management of a patient in coma is described in Chapter 1. After head injury it is especially important to monitor carefully the patient's neurological status because deterioration due to intracranial haemorrhage may develop rapidly. Neurological observations should be made at 15-minute intervals until there is definite evidence of improvement or stabilization. Patients with severe head injury may remain in coma for many weeks, often on a life-support machine. The long-term management of such cases is beyond the scope of this book, but from the outset expert nursing, anaesthetic care and regular physiotherapy are necessary. Chest infection, seizures and metabolic imbalance are all common and considerably complicate management and neurological assessment. It should not be forgotten, however, that even after prolonged periods of coma good recovery is possible.

Anticonvulsant treatment should be started in comatose patients with a depressed fracture or intracranial haemorrhage and in those who have had seizures. A 1000-mg loading dose of phenytoin should be given either IV over 30 minutes or orally over 24 hours (see page 86 for details), followed by a maintenance dose of 300 mg/day adjusted according to serum levels. Prophylactic anticonvulsants are probably not indicated in other patients. Broad-spectrum antibiotic treatment should be given to patients with a depressed fracture or those with a basal fracture complicated by leakage of CSF or blood from the nose or ear, and relevant swabs should be taken for culture.

THE CONSCIOUS PATIENT

After admission regular neurological observations should be made. If the head injury was mild and there is no sign of deterioration, the patient may be discharged after 12–24 hours with a written instruction sheet. Mild analgesics should be used to control headache; opiates and other major analgesics or sedative drugs should be avoided as they may complicate subsequent neurological assessment.

TRANSFER TO OR CONSULTATION WITH NEUROSURGICAL DEPARTMENT

A telephone consultation should be made with the neurosurgical department whenever the physician in charge requires advice. Absolute criteria are difficult to give, but one should not feel diffident about seeking advice when faced with an acutely ill patient and transfer, if required, should be carried out as soon as possible. The criteria of the Department of Neurosurgery of the Institute of Neurological Sciences, Glasgow, UK, are presented in Table 6.3. Transfer to a neurosurgical unit should always be made with personnel able to insert or re-position an endotracheal tube and initiate or maintain ventilation.

*Table 6.3 Criteria for considering transfer to neurosurgical unit**

Fractured skull with confusion or impairment of consciousness, seizures or focal symptoms or signs
Coma continuing after resuscitation
Deteriorating level of consciousness
Developing neurological signs
Confusion or drowsiness persisting for >6–8 h
Compound depressed fracture of the skull vault
Suspected fracture of the skull base (e.g. with CSF rhinorrhoea, otorrhoea, bilateral orbital haematoma, mastoid haematoma)
Penetrating injury

*Patients in the first four categories should be referred urgently. In all cases the diagnosis and initial treatment of serious extracranial injury should take priority over transfer to a neurosurgical unit. (Derived from guidelines of the Department of Neurosurgery, Institute of Neurological Sciences, Glasgow, UK.)

IMMEDIATE COMPLICATIONS

LACERATION AND OPEN HEAD INJURY

Lacerations are important: they may indicate the site of a skull fracture, act as a source of infection, and be the site of significant blood loss. All lacerations should be shaved for 3 cm around the wound and inspected thoroughly before cleaning and suturing.

LINEAR SKULL FRACTURE

Specific treatment is not usually required if this occurs over the vault. Basal fractures may cause bleeding or CSF leakage through the ear or the sinuses; broad-spectrum antibiotic cover is necessary if this occurs. Usually the leak is self-limiting, but the patient should remain under observation in hospital until it has stopped.

DEPRESSED SKULL FRACTURE

If a depressed skull fracture is seen on X-ray or is obvious clinically, neurosurgical treatment is usually required and the patient should be transferred to a neurosurgical unit. There is a risk of meningitis or cerebral infection and broad-spectrum antibiotics are necessary. Epilepsy is also a common sequela and prophylactic anticonvulsant treatment should be initiated. A depressed fracture may be easily missed, particularly if it affects the paranasal sinuses, and radiography needs to be of high quality.

ACUTE EXTRADURAL HAEMORRHAGE

This is usually caused by tearing of the middle meningeal arteries due to fracture of the skull across their course. As the blood is under arterial pressure, extradural haematomas may collect rapidly and the patient is often unconscious upon arrival at hospital. Although there is commonly a *lucid interval* of minutes or hours between the initial injury and subsequent rapid deterioration, this does not always occur. The signs of an extradural haemorrhage are initially those of focal neurological disturbance, followed by those of rapidly rising intracranial pressure and, finally, those of transtentorial herniation (coning) (see page 14).

Often the focal deficits are barely noticed as events proceed rapidly, but the development of a progressive hemiparesis or dysphasia after a head injury requires immediate action. The predominant signs of raised intracranial pressure are headache, drowsiness and coma. By the time the signs of coning have developed, irreparable brain damage may have occurred. This is an acute emergency. The patient should be given IV mannitol and surgical removal of the haematoma should be undertaken

Immediate Complications 67

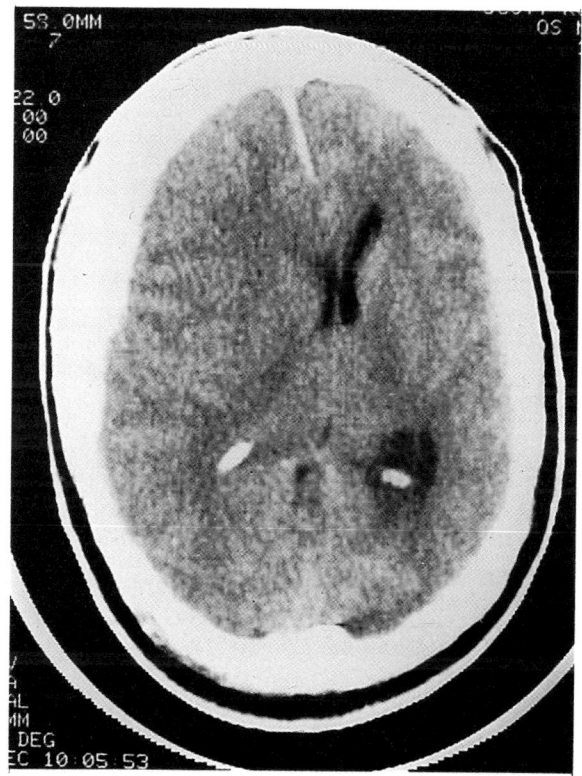

Figure 6.1 CT showing extradural haematoma. Kindly donated by Dr G. Tatler.

immediately. There is often no time to arrange neurosurgical transfer; hence, the emergency is usually dealt with by the general surgical team. An extradural haematoma can be diagnosed firmly by CT (Fig. 6.1) but this may take too long to organize and surgical intervention is often necessary on the basis of a presumptive clinical diagnosis, perhaps supported by radiological evidence of a fracture crossing the course of the middle meningeal artery. Prophylactic anticonvulsant therapy (Chapter 8) should be instituted before surgery.

ACUTE SUBDURAL HAEMORRHAGE

This is caused by bleeding into the subdural space, usually

68 Head Injury

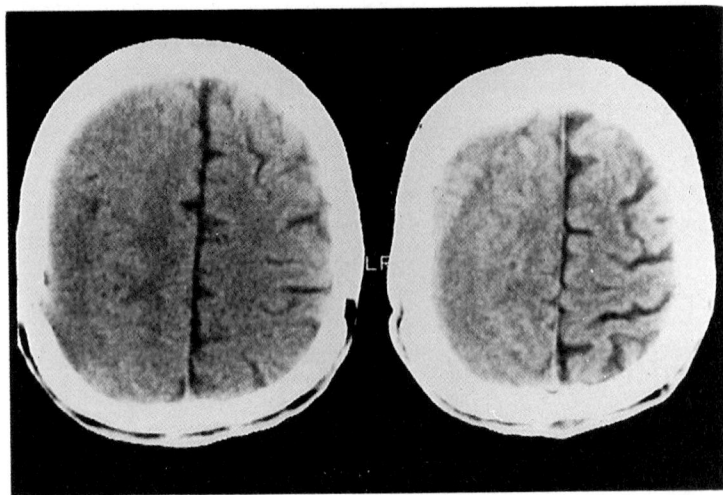

Figure 6.2 CT showing subdural haematoma. Kindly donated by Dr G. Tatler.

from tearing of vessels in the region of the sylvian fissure. The clinical presentation may be similar to that of acute extradural haemorrhage or less rapidly progressive. Diagnosis is made clinically or with CT (Fig. 6.2) and immediate surgical decompression is vital. IV mannitol (200 mls of a 20% solution over 10 minutes) and prophylactic anticonvulsant cover (IM phenobarbitone or IV phenytoin) can be given while arrangements are being made for CT or surgery.

ACUTE INTRACEREBRAL HAEMORRHAGE

This is another ominous complication of head injury. Haemorrhage occurs most commonly in the frontal and temporal lobes. The clinical presentation depends on the size of the haematoma and the associated brain swelling, and management depends on the severity and progression of the neurological disturbance. IV corticosteroid therapy (dexamethasone, 4–10 mg, 6-hourly) should be instituted if there is any evidence of raised intracranial pressure; IV mannitol (50–100 g) should be used if pressure is critically raised or in preparation for surgery. The surgical evacuation of a haemorrhage is necessary in selected patients only, and an urgent specialist neurological consultation should be arranged. Whether or not surgical treatment is carried out, it is advisable to provide prophylactic anticonvulsant cover.

The main reason for making regular neurological observations on a patient after head injury is to detect quickly the signs of intracranial haemorrhage. It must be made clear to the nursing staff that signs of deterioration require *immediate* notification. Too often, observations are made and deterioration noted but no action taken.

POST-TRAUMATIC SEIZURES

Epileptic seizures, and occasionally status epilepticus, occur in about five per cent of those admitted to hospital with head injury. In the acute phase they may indicate an intracranial haemorrhage and CT should be carried out. Immediate anticonvulsant therapy should be instituted with IV diazepam and phenytoin as outlined on page 85.

CRANIAL NERVE INJURY

This often occurs after severe head injury. The olfactory, facial and oculomotor nerves are most commonly affected. Radiology may show a fracture in the relevant position. The deficit should be recorded for medico-legal purposes, but there is no specific treatment. The importance to the emergency setting is that a peripheral lesion may be confused with focal cerebral or brain stem damage or with incipient coning. However, the oculomotor defects due to coning occur in the context of rapidly rising intracranial pressure and the diagnosis should be clinically obvious.

INAPPROPRIATE ADH SECRETION

This may develop quickly after head injury, resulting in an apparent neurological deterioration with confusion or drowsiness. Diagnosis, which is straightforward, is made by the finding of hyponatraemia and low serum urea with a low plasma and high urinary osmolality. Treatment is by fluid restriction.

OTHER INJURY

Often a patient with severe head trauma has sustained other orthopaedic or abdominal injuries, and it is important not to overlook these. Significant blood loss may also occur, contributing to the drowsiness or coma.

FURTHER READING

Jennett B, Teasdale G.
Management of Head Injuries. Philadelphia: FA Davis, 1981.

Fonton Lewis A, ed.
Harrogate Seminar Report No. 8: The Management of Acute Head Injury. London: Department of Health and Society Security, 1983.

7. Acute spinal cord dysfunction

The spinal cord stretches from the base of the skull to the level of the first lumbar vertebra in the adult, and may be damaged acutely anywhere along its course by either intrinsic or extrinsic disease. As is the case throughout the central nervous system, established neurological damage is usually irreversible but there is often a period in the acute phase when recovery is possible. For this reason, and to prevent the spread of any damage, acute spinal cord dysfunction requires urgent attention. Early diagnosis and treatment may prevent permanent disabling neurological deficit. The clinical history and examination usually enable identification of the level of the cord lesion, but the pathological diagnosis may require specialized investigation.

CLINICAL FEATURES OF SPINAL CORD DYSFUNCTION

Regardless of cause the clinical features of acute spinal cord conditions can be summarized as follows.

SPINAL PAIN
This is common both in space-occupying lesions (e.g. malignant or benign tumours), when it is often present for some time before neurological dysfunction develops, and in trauma. It may be confined to the area of the lesion or spread as root pain; in either case it is of great localizing value. There may also be local tenderness to percussion.

MOTOR SIGNS
Weakness may be of lower motor neuron type at the level of the lesion (i.e. in the arm in cervical cord lesions) and

Table 7.1 Motor weakness in spinal cord dysfunction

Lower motor neuron weakness[*]	Upper motor neuron weakness[†]
Flaccid tone	Spastic tone
Hyporeflexia	Hyperreflexia
Wasting (in chronic cases)	Weakness in pyramidal distribution[‡]
Weakness in root distribution	

[*]Due to root or anterior horn cell damage at the level of the lesion.
[†]Due to damage of the corticospinal tracts supplying muscles below the level of the lesion.
In the acute phase of an injury the tone may be flaccid and reflexes absent or reduced even with upper motor neuron damage (the phase of spinal shock).
[‡]Weakness of the extensor muscles of upper limbs and flexor muscles of lower limbs.

pyramidal (upper motor neuron) below the level of the lesion (Table 7.1). The pyramidal weakness is usually *bilateral* but not necessarily symmetrical, and this is a very useful way of differentiating the weakness in lesions of the spinal cord and cerebral hemispheres.

SENSORY SIGNS

Alteration of limb sensation may be of several types depending on the part of the cord affected (Fig. 7.1). A sensory level may be detectable on the trunk and should always be carefully sought as it is a very useful diagnostic sign and helpful in localizing the site of damage. A true sensory level can occur (with rare exceptions) only in spinal cord disease, is higher on the back than on the ventral surface and found at or just below the level of the lesion.

SPHINCTERIC SIGNS

Impairment of micturition and/or sexual function usually occurs before alteration of bowel function. Examination of the patient should always include a careful assessment of bladder enlargement, which may be painless because of concurrent sensory loss.

Clinical Features 73

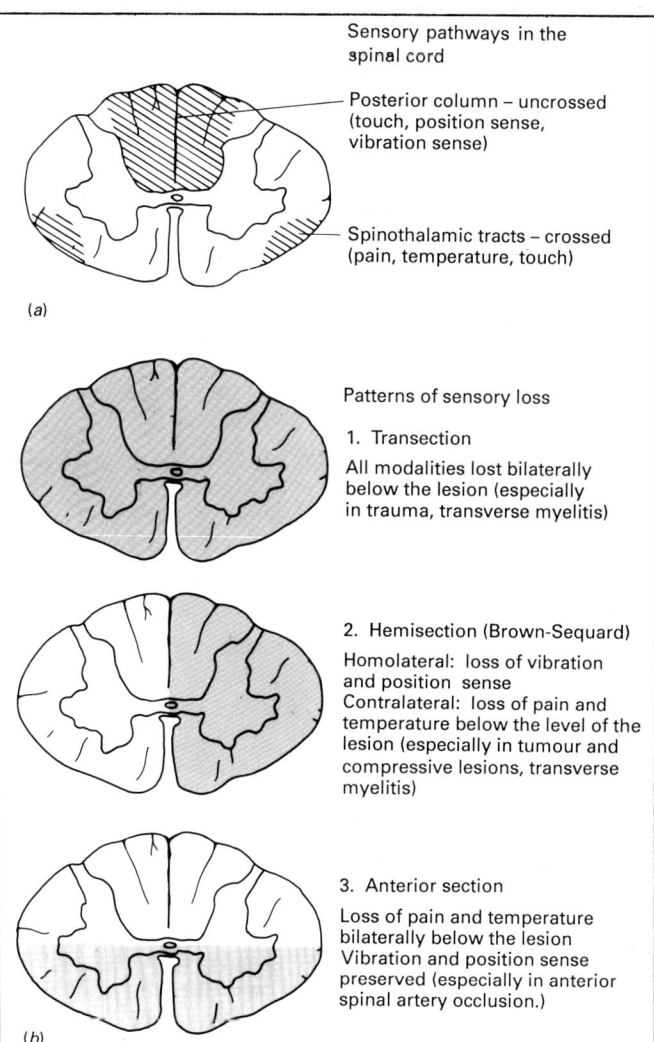

Figure 7.1 Sensory disturbance in spinal disease.

RESPIRATORY SIGNS

In patients with high cervical lesions the diaphragm (supplied by segments C2-C4) may be weak and respiratory failure may ensue. Respiratory distress requires urgent action (Chapter 9).

74 Acute Spinal Cord Dysfunction

Table 7.2 Causes of acute spinal cord compression

Tumour	Infection	Degenerative spinal disease	Other
Metastatic	Pyogenic spinal abscess	Cervical spondylosis	Paget's disease of bone
Primary extradural intradural	Parasitic cyst	Prolapsed intra-vertebral disc	Arachnoiditis
Myeloma			Arachnoid cyst
Reticulosis			Epidural haematoma
			Congenital bony abnormalities

Especially from breast, prostate, lung.
Especially sarcoma, chrodoma, haemangioblastoma.
Especially meningioma, neurofibroma, ependymoma, astrocytoma.
Especially staphylococcal or tuberculous.
e.g. craniocervical abnormalities, kyphoscoliosis, achondroplasia.

ACUTE SPINAL CORD COMPRESSION

Spinal cord compression may be acute, subacute or chronic (Table 7.2). In chronic cases the early symptoms may be slight or insignificant, and it is surprising how often marked weakness, alteration in sensation or impairment of sphincteric function are initially ignored by both the patient and physician. Chronic compression may suddenly deteriorate, and present as an acute emergency. The symptoms and signs are those of spinal cord dysfunction (see above). Although specific lesions tend to exhibit characteristic symptom-complexes, these are seldom diagnostic.

METASTATIC TUMOUR

This is one of the commonest causes of cord compression. Pain is a prominent feature and there is usually evidence of malignancy elsewhere: carcinoma of breast, lung or prostate, lymphoma and myeloma are most frequently encountered. Plain radiology is often diagnostic, emergency corticosteroid therapy (dexamethasone, 4–10 mg, 6-hourly) is often helpful, urgent radiotherapy should be considered and immediate surgical decompression may produce dramatic improvement in neurological function and relieve pain.

PRIMARY TUMOUR

These are usually slow-growing and although symptoms might have been present for some time, acute deterioration in neurological status may occur. The commonest are neurofibroma (which may have been present for months or years before cord symptoms develop and characteristically causes root pain at the level of the lesion), meningioma, haemangioblastoma and ependymoma. Diagnosis is made by plain radiography and myelography. Treatment is surgical.

INFECTION

Spinal epidural abscess is an important and potentially treatable cause of cord compression and can result from bacterial (especially *Staphylococcus aureus* and *Mycobacterium tuberculosis*), fungal or parasitic infection. There are usually but not always signs of systemic infection. A spinal abscess is usually very painful. Plain radiography is occasionally normal. Urgent surgical drainage and antibiotic therapy are necessary.

DISC DISEASE

Herniation of an intravertebral disc is usually lateral, causing symptoms of root compression; rarely, however, a central herniation will occur and result in cord compression, particularly in the thoracic region (where the spinal canal is narrowest) and in congenitally narrow canals. It may also be precipitated by trauma. Permanent cord damage may ensue and this, unlike most 'disc disease', is a medical emergency. Diagnosis is made by plain radiology (thoracic discs are often calcified and the disc space narrowed) and myelography. Treatment is by immediate surgical decompression.

DEGENERATIVE SPINAL COLUMN DISEASE

Spondylosis, particularly in the cervical region, may cause symptomatic cord compression. The disability is often compounded by concurrent vascular damage. Diagnosis is made by plain radiology and myelography. Immobilization is often the most useful emergency measure, but treatment may be difficult.

EPIDURAL HAEMATOMA

This may occur spontaneously in patients with coagulation defects or on anticoagulant therapy (and has been reported after lumbar puncture in anticoagulated patients) or can be due to haemangioma or angioma of the cord or spinal column. Diagnosis is made by myelography. Immediate surgical decompression is usually indicated.

ACUTE NON-COMPRESSIVE SPINAL CORD LESIONS

The most important causes (Table 7.3) are as follows.

ACUTE TRANSVERSE MYELITIS

This may occur in a number of conditions but in over half the cases no aetiological diagnosis is made. The syndrome is a common manifestation of multiple sclerosis or other demyelinating diseases. The clinical features are those of a painless cord lesion and may progress over a matter of hours or days. The CSF often shows a lymphocytic pleocytosis, moderate elevation of protein, depending on the cause, and other specific features. In many cases the diagnosis can only be made after myelography has excluded a compressive lesion.

VASCULAR INFARCTION

Occasionally, infarction of the cord will occur due to lesions

Table 7.3 Causes of acute non-compressive spinal cord lesions

Acute transverse myelitis	Vascular infarction	Other
Multiple sclerosis (and Devic's disease)	Anterior spinal artery syndrome: arteriosclerotic hypotension embolic aortic dissection postoperative	Toxins
		Drugs
Acute disseminated encephalomyelitis		Vitamin deficiency
		Radiation
Postinfective (immunologically based)	Spinal angioma	Decompression sickness
Postvaccination	Vasculitis (e.g. collagen disease, PAN)	Syringomyelia
Viral myelitis (e.g. herpes zoster)	Sickle cell	AIDS
Syphilitic	Cervical myelopathy in cervical spondylosis	
Sarcoidosis	Trauma	

of the anterior spinal artery. Damage is maximal in the thoracic region. Generalized atheroma is the usual cause although the syndrome may be produced by severe hypotension (especially during surgery), intra-arterial embolism, dissection of the descending aorta (or interference during aortic surgery), vasculitis, sickle cell disease or spinal angioma. The condition presents with an acute, painless, often severe weakness of the legs, paralysis of sphincteric function and alteration of sensation to pinprick and light touch, with preservation of vibration and position sense (as the vascular insult is maximal ventrally in the cord and the posterior columns are spared). Radiology will be normal. The CSF may be normal or show a mild leucocytosis. Treatment is symptomatic.

CERVICAL SPONDYLOSIS

Even in the absence of compression this may cause a myelopathy due to vascular insufficiency. An acute deterioration (e.g. precipitated in mild trauma) may present as an emergency in patients with a previous chronic myelopathy. The vascular damage in cervical spondylosis, unlike that in anterior spinal artery disease, may affect any part of the cervical cord, affecting all sensory modalities.

OTHER CAUSES

These are numerous and include vitamin deficiency, iatrogenic disease (particularly intrathecal drug therapy), radiation, AIDS and toxins. Chronic spinal cord disease, such as subacute combined degeneration of the cord, syringomyelia or tabes dorsalis, may also worsen acutely.

EMERGENCY MANAGEMENT IN ACUTE SPINAL CORD DYSFUNCTION

In most cases the site of the lesion can be established by clinical and radiological examination, and its pathology determined from the clinical history and investigations. The following plan should be adopted in all cases of acute spinal cord dysfunction.

1. Undertake careful clinical examination (general and neurological), including full motor and sensory testing.

2. Assess respiratory function (especially in cervical cord damage) and, if this is impaired, the need for artificial respiration (Chapter 9).

3. Assess sphincteric function and catheterize the bladder if its function is impaired.

4. Assess skin for pressure sores etc. and arrange for careful nursing of patients with paralysed limbs.

5. Arrange for immediate plain antero-posterior, lateral and oblique X-ray views of the affected region.

6. Spinal cord compression: consider myelography in all

cases for whom compression is a possibility. Myelography may be required in an emergency (at night if necessary) if the compression is critical, as indicated by impairment of sphincteric function, leg weakness so severe that the patient is unable to stand or rapidly progressive neurological deficit. In such cases even a delay of hours can result in serious, permanent neurological disability. An urgent neurological or neurosurgical opinion should be sought in all cases of cord compression. If possible, the neurological assessment should be made before myelography, which can worsen the patient's condition.

7. Non-compressive spinal cord diseases: if the suspicion of an acute myelitis is high, lumbar puncture, which may be confirmatory, should be performed. Often, however, the possibility of compression cannot be excluded and myelography is usually necessary if there is any doubt. This may be technically more difficult if a prior lumbar puncture has been carried out.

8. Empirical therapy with corticosteroids (dexamethasone, 4–10 mg, 6-hourly, initially IV then orally) may reduce swelling in critical cases of spinal cord compression, especially in malignant disease, abscess or in acute transverse myelitis.

ACUTE SPINAL CORD INJURY

Trauma is a common cause of spinal cord damage. In major trauma it is very easy to overlook spinal column injury as its clinical manifestations may be less dramatic than those of other neurological, orthopaedic or abdominal injuries. It is important to remember this, however, as manipulation of an unstable spine may result in cord damage and permanent neurological damage. In a case of possible spinal column injury, the following procedure should be followed.

EMERGENCY ASSESSMENT

Neurological
The degree of neurological damage should first be assessed. If the patient is conscious, sensory and motor function in the extremities should be tested. Neck and back pain, and limitation of movement should be assessed. Even in an emergency, motor power, reflexes and sensation to pin-prick and vibration should be tested and, if circumstances permit, a more comprehensive neurological examination carried out. If no abnormality is present at this stage, then spinal cord function is intact. If a neurological deficit is found, the level should be identified clinically.

Orthopaedic
It is vital to determine whether the spine is stable or unstable. This will usually only be possible after a radiological examination.

Respiratory function
This may be impaired in upper cervical cord damage. Any sign of respiratory embarrassment should be treated immediately.

MOVEMENT OF THE PATIENT
If neurological abnormalities are present or the spinal column is potentially unstable, some sort of spinal brace should be applied, ideally at the scene of the accident, before the patient is moved. However, even after the patient has arrived at the casualty department, further mishandling may —and, sadly, frequently does — cause irreversible spinal cord damage. Support should take the form of a stiff collar, strapping to a stretcher or backboard, and/or immobilization with sandbags as circumstances dictate. Great care should be taken in any movement of the patient, particularly an unconscious patient.

RADIOLOGICAL DIAGNOSIS
Radiological examination is essential in all cases of spinal

injury to assess the type, extent, severity and stability of the bony injury. Reasonable quality antero-posterior lateral and oblique X-rays are usually required. Additional views to show the position of the odontoid peg may be necessary. Great care must be taken when moving the patient on the X-ray table.

OTHER MEASURES

1. Blood pressure should be carefully maintained as hypotension may worsen neurological damage in spinal injury. High cervical injury may itself cause hypotension, but it is usually the result of blood loss or abdominal injury.

2. Sphincteric function should be assessed; catheterization of the bladder may be necessary.

3. Skin care and care of the paralysed limbs should be instituted immediately.

4. Dexamethasone therapy (4–10 mg, 6-hourly, initially IV) may be given if there is severe neurological impairment, although there is little firm evidence it confers any benefit.

OTHER COMPLICATIONS

Other injuries should be identified. These are usually obvious (it is often the spinal injury that is most likely to be overlooked) but in the presence of spinal damage sensory loss may result in intra-abdominal injuries being painless and peritoneal signs minimal.

TREATMENT

If spinal injury is confirmed or suspected, transfer for immediate neurological or orthopaedic care is imperative. Myelography, permanent traction or surgical fixation may be necessary but the indications for these depend on the stability of the spine and the extent of neurological involvement. Decisions regarding these specific measures should be taken by an experienced surgeon.

8. Status Epilepticus

Status epilepticus is best defined as recurring seizures without recovery of consciousness for 30 minutes or more. Classification is usually made according to the International Classification of Epileptic Seizures. Convulsive status is the only common 'medical emergency' in this group and discussion will be limited to this condition. Pseudoseizures commonly present as "status", and are often misdiagnosed in the emergency setting.

Convulsive status epilepticus may develop in the course of established epilepsy (60%) or as the initial (15%) or only (25%) epileptic manifestation. Idiopathic epilepsy rarely presents as status in adult life; the onset of status therefore implies an acute underlying cause (Table 8.1). The site of the cerebral pathology is also important; frontal lobe lesions such as trauma or tumour are more likely to produce status epilepticus than are lesions in other parts of the brain. About 1%–5% of patients with established epilepsy at some time develop status for which there is usually a precipitating cause (Table 8.2).

Convulsive status epilepticus is a serious condition with a mortality rate of 5%–25% even with adequate treatment. There is also significant morbidity (e.g. focal neurological damage, intellectual decline, behavioural changes, continuing epilepsy). The rates of morbidity and mortality

Table 8.1 Aetiology in cases of status epilepticus presenting in adults without a history of epilepsy

Trauma	20%
Tumour	20%
Encephalitis	10%
Vascular	10%
Miscellaneous	20%
No cause found	20%

Table 8.2 Precipitating causes of status in established epilepsy

Poor anticonvulsant compliance/sudden drug withdrawal	25%
Alcohol	10%
Intercurrent infection	10%
Miscellaneous (e.g. drugs, pregnancy, vascular events)	10%
Unknown	45%

are higher in children and patients with structural brain lesions. The longer the status continues, the worse the prognosis. Status may cause brain damage as a direct result of hypoxia, hypoglycaemia, hyperpyrexia, hypotension or other metabolic disturbances (e.g. acidosis, changes in calcium levels) but how much of the morbidity is due to these direct effects, inappropriate drug therapy or medical complications is often unclear. There is no doubt, however, that both the mortality and morbidity of the condition are minimized by effective initial emergency treatment.

EMERGENCY MANAGEMENT

RESUSCITATION

The principles of resuscitation in status are similar to those in other neurological emergencies. In the acute stages emphasis should be placed on the maintenance of cardiorespiratory function and circulation (Chapter 9). Particular attention should be directed towards the following.

IV line

The setting up of a secure IV line is often difficult in a patient who is fitting, and may have to wait until an initial bolus dose of diazepam has been given (see below). Many anticonvulsant drugs cause severe phlebitis, so it is important to choose a large vein. Saline, not glucose, should be infused. The drugs should not be given intra-arterially.

Protection of cardiorespiratory function

Because of the increased metabolic activity caused by active convulsions and the depressant effect of anticonvulsant drugs, there is a particular risk of cardiorespiratory insufficiency. In all cases oxygen should be administered immediately via a mask or intratracheal tube because hypoxia is common and its extent is usually underestimated.

Sudden respiratory collapse may occur; hence, it is best to intubate and institute artificial respiration sooner rather than later in the course of a prolonged episode.

Thiamine and glucose
Thiamine (50 mg IV and 50 mg IM) and glucose (50 mg IV of 50% glucose solution) should be given immediately if there is any suspicion of alcoholism or hypoglycaemia, both of which may present as seizures.

EMERGENCY INVESTIGATIONS
A 50 ml sample of venous blood should be taken immediately and rapid estimations made of anticonvulsant levels (if appropriate), full blood count, urea, electrolytes, sugar, calcium and magnesium levels. Arterial blood gases should be estimated if there is any suggestion of hypoxia or if artificial ventilation is to be instituted. Metabolic abnormalities may be the cause of the status or may develop during its course and treatment. Other investigations (e.g. CT scanning, blood culture, lumbar puncture) depend on clinical circumstances.

AETIOLOGY AND PRECIPITATING FACTORS
The cause of the seizures or the precipitating factors should be established as soon as possible. The history is of paramount importance in this respect. First, it is important to ascertain whether the patient has a history of epilepsy because the causes of status in such cases differ from those in patients without previous epilepsy (Tables 8.1 and 8.2). In a patient with known epilepsy the immediate precipitating factors should be determined. In a patient without previous epilepsy enquiries should concentrate on any preceding illness, including any history of infection, head injury, raised intracranial pressure, etc. It should not be forgotten that complications can develop in patients with established epilepsy who may, for instance, sustain subdural haemorrhages or have previously undetected cerebral tumours. Patients should be examined neurologically for focal signs and signs of raised intracranial pressure. A general examination may reveal a Medi-Alert bracelet, signs

of infection, head injury, etc.

MEDICAL COMPLICATIONS

A number of complications may develop as a direct result of recurrent seizures (Table 8.3) and every effort should be made to detect and treat them.

ANTICONVULSANT THERAPY

This should be given to achieve immediate suppression of seizures and provide long-term anticonvulsant protection (Table 8.4). If the second is neglected, as all too often is the case, seizures will recur quickly after initial suppression and may be more difficult to control subsequently.

Immediate seizure control

Discussion will be limited to diazepam, phenytoin, chlormethiazole and paraldehyde, as these are sufficient for the initial management of most cases; for refractory cases, there are other preparations that may become necessary at a later stage (see below).

Diazepam. In adults 10–20 mg diazepam should be administered IV or given rectally (as a solution, not as a suppository) (Table 8.5). This dosage may be repeated at

---

Table 8.3 Medical complications of status epilepticus

Respiratory failure and hypoxia
Cardiovascular collapse
Pulmonary oedema
Pulmonary embolism
Hypo/hypertension
Cardiac arrhythmia
Infection (especially chest)
Dehydration
Hyperthermia
Metabolic disturbance[*]
DIC
Orthopaedic injury

---

[*]e.g. hypoglycaemia; hypocalcaemia; electrolyte, hepatic, or renal disturbance.

Table 8.4 Emergency anticonvulsant treatment

Immediate control	Longer-term control
IV Diazepam (or IM paraldehyde)	If already on anticonvulsant drugs, continue via NG tube
If this fails, IV phenytoin or IV chlormethiazole (in sequence)	If not, phenytoin via NG tube, then carbamazepine or valproate if necessary
If this fails, IV thiopentone	

intervals of 10 minutes or more, to a maximum of 50 mg in 4 hours. Often, diazepam (with or without paraldehyde) has already been administered before the patient is seen in casualty; if the dosage has already exceeded the above limits phenytoin treatment should be started immediately (see below). It is essential to monitor respiration during the administration of diazepam and facilities for immediate resuscitation should be available if >20 mg is to be given. Diazepam is often all that is needed to control the seizures. However, even if seizures are arrested the patient should be kept under observation for at least another 6 hours. If the seizures are not suppressed, arrangements must be made for immediate admission, if necessary, to an intensive care unit.

The significant side-effects of diazepam in patients with status are respiratory depression (which may develop quickly and unexpectedly), depression of consciousness and, rarely, hypotension. Some deaths due to status epilepticus are caused by the injudicious use of diazepam. As diazepam is metabolized in the liver, it should be used cautiously in patients with liver failure although, initially at least, the dose need not be altered. No dosage adjustments are necessary in cases of renal failure.

If IV diazepam fails to control the seizures or they recur after an initial response to diazepam, an infusion of phenytoin or chlormethiazole should be started immediately.

Phenytoin. In adults a loading dose of 1000 mg (in a saline, not glucose, drip) should be given (via an infusion pump if

Table 8.5 Anticonvulsants in status epilepticus in adults

Anticonvulsant	Indications	Dosage and administration	Peak cerebral levels	Side-effects
Diazepam	Initial therapy (given IV or rectally)	10–20 mg boluses at 1–5 mg/min, repeated to max. of 50 mg/4 h (separate doses by at least 10 min)	IV <1 min Rectal <4 min	Respiratory depression Depression of consciousness
Phenytoin	After diazepam	IV loading dose: 1000 mg into a large vein, max. of 50 mg/min (i.e. over 20–30 min); in a saline, not glucose, drip; monitor ECG	15–20 min	Hypotension and cardiovascular collapse Cardiac arrhythmia
Chlormethiazole	After diazepam and/or phenytoin		15–30 min	Hypotension and cardiovascular collapse Mild respiratory depression
Paraldehyde	Where IV therapy not possible or resuscitation facilities unavailable	IV/oral maintenance dose: 100mg, 6-hourly (begin IV 6h after loading dose; oral, as soon as possible, given as above)	<30 min	Depression of consciousness

IV bolus of 100 ml over 5–10 min, repeated over 5–10 min if necessary and followed by an infusion of 4–10 ml/min (60–150 drops/min) titrating dose against response; given in a 0.8% solution (usually already made up)	Thrombophlebitis Depression of consciousness Respiratory depression∗
5–10 ml deep IM injection, repeated every 2–4 h if necessary; 4–5mls PR, as a 10% enema in isotonic saline	Hypotension and cardiovascular collapse Pulmonary oedema Apnoea Pain at injection site Sterile abscess

possible) at a rate not exceeding 50 mg/min (i.e. over 20–30 min) (Table 8.5). It is imperative to monitor carefully the ECG for cardiac arrhythmia during the infusion. A therapeutic blood level of phenytoin will normally be achieved within 30 minutes of the onset of infusion and maintained for at least 12 hours. After the first infusion phenytoin should be given as a 100-mg bolus in a saline drip every 6 hours (over 2 or more min) although it may be necessary to make dosage adjustments according to the serum levels.

The major side-effects of phenytoin are cardiac arrhythmia, hypotension and, less commonly, respiratory depression and depression of consciousness. These depend more on the rate of administration than on the total dose and are rare if the rate is kept <50 mg/min. As phenytoin is metabolized in the liver, it should be used cautiously in patients with liver failure although, as with diazepam, no initial dosage adjustments are necessary. Similarly, no dosage adjustments are needed in cases of renal failure; however, as phenytoin is highly protein-bound, total serum levels may be unreliable in uraemic patients with altered plasma proteins, necessitating measurement of free plasma levels.

Chlormethiazole. This should be given IV as a 0.8% solution (Table 8.5). In the UK chlormethiazole (Heminervin) is supplied already made up to this concentration. Initially, a bolus of 100 ml should be given over 5–10 minutes. If the seizures stop this initial dosage can be reduced. The infusion is then continued at a dose of 4–10 ml/min as required (60–150 drops/min). The advantage of this drug is its very short half-life (2–5 h) and very quick onset of action (within 3–5 min); thus, the dose can be adjusted according to the clinical response.

Side-effects of chlormethiazole include thrombophlebitis, nasal tingling, sneezing, pulmonary oedema (usually mild) and depressed consciousness. It has relatively few cardiorespiratory complications although it may potentiate the effects of other sedative drugs. Over a prolonged period it may degrade plastic tubing.

Paraldehyde. If IV drug administration is not possible or facilities for resuscitation are not available, IM or rectal paraldehyde may be used as an initial therapy for status epilepticus (Table 8.5). A deep IM injection of 5 ml should be given into each buttock, repeated every 2–4 hours if necessary. Paraldehyde is rapidly absorbed and acts quickly (peak plasma levels are obtained <30 min). It is often effective as an initial treatment, but if seizures continue, transfer to a setting where IV therapy is possible should be arranged. There is little place for IM paraldehyde after diazepam, phenytoin or chlormethiazole. Paraldehyde may also by given rectally (4–5 mls, administered as a 10% enema in isotonic saline).

Paraldehyde is difficult to use: as it reacts with plastic, it must be injected from a glass syringe. It decomposes rapidly in the light; hence, the contents of an opened container must be used within 24 hours. It may cause hypotension and cardiovascular collapse but these are rare and probably due to poor dilution or decomposition of the drug. Pulmonary oedema and, more rarely, apnoea may occur. It should be given as a deep IM injection, which is very painful, and if administered injudiciously can result in severe sciatic nerve damage or a sterile abscess at the injection site.

Long-term seizure control

It should be established whether or not the patient is currently receiving anticonvulsant drugs. If so it is vital that these should be continued as soon as possible, regardless of other emergency treatment, via a naso-gastric tube if necessary. Anticonvulsant levels should be measured prior to this and the dosage adjusted to obtain levels in the upper therapeutic range. If the patient was not on medication prior to the episode of status, an oral loading dose of 500 mg phenytoin should be administered (if an IV loading dose has not been given), and repeated after 6 hours and followed by 100 mg, orally, 6-hourly. Alternatively, carbamazepine or valproate can be administered.

Intramuscular drug administration

It is essential to emphasize that, with the exception of paraldehyde and phenobarbitone, no anticonvulsant should ever be given IM as this will often further complicate an already serious clinical situation. The drugs are erratically, insufficiently and slowly absorbed after IM administration, which may interfere with subsequent drug treatment. Phenytoin, for instance, may achieve a level of less than 5 µmol/l after 24 hours and cause local damage at the injection site. IM medication is often given in a belief, which is wholly mistaken, that an IM injection must be better than nothing!

REFRACTORY STATUS EPILEPTICUS

If the above measures do not control the status, the patient should be transferred to an ITU, intubated and artificial ventilation instituted. It may be necessary to proceed to treatment with thiopentone if the seizures continue relentlessly. Thiopentone is given as a 100–200 mg bolus dose, followed by 50 mg doses every 3 minutes until epileptic activity ceases, and then as a constant infusion (via a pump if possible) of 125 mg/h. As thiopentone has a relatively short half-life its effects can be quickly reversed. This is important as there is a serious possibility of cardiovascular depression with prolonged usage. It may be necessary to monitor the central venous pressure or pulmonary capillary wedge pressure.

EEG monitoring is advisable in all cases of refractory epilepsy and is particularly important in anaesthetized, paralysed and ventilated patients as it may be the only way of detecting epileptic activity.

Other IV anticonvulsant drugs may be tried if the above fail to control the seizures fully. These include phenobarbitone, clonazepam, lorazepam and steroids, but they are not discussed further here because by the time their use is contemplated the patient should be in specialist hands.

If seizures continue despite initial treatment, it is important to reassess carefully the clinical circumstances because there are often complicating factors that may require urgent action and will otherwise prolong or worsen the epilepsy. These include the following.

1. Inadequate anticonvulsant treatment which is perhaps the commonest cause.

2. Hypoxia, which is frequent and often overlooked. Estimation of blood gases is mandatory and oxygen should be administered routinely in all cases of status.

3. Metabolic disturbances, especially acidosis, hypocalcaemia and hypoglycaemia. A full biochemical screen must be carried out urgently; such disturbances may have developed during the course of treatment or may have been the initial cause of the status.

4. Failure to detect the underlying cause of the epilepsy. This is particularly relevant with progressive cerebral lesions (e.g. infection, haemorrhage).

5. Other medical complications (e.g. hyperthermia, cardiorespiratory problems).

6. Diagnosis incorrect, and patient exhibiting pseudoseizures.

Table 8.6 Anticonvulsants: adjustment of dosages for children

Anticonvulsant Initial loading dose

Anticonvulsant	Initial loading dose
Diazepam	IV bolus: 0.3–0.5 mg/kg or 1 mg/yr of age + 1 mg Rectal: 0.5 mg/kg
Phenytoin*	IV: 10–15 mg/kg over 30 min, not exceeding 50 mg/min
Chlormethizole	IV: 0.01 ml 0.8% solution/kg/min, increasing to a max. of 0.1 ml/kg/min
Paraldehyde	IV: 1 ml/yr of age, up to max. of 5 ml

*IV/oral maintenance dose: 100–200 mg/day (up to 7 yr), as for adult >7 yr

DRUG TREATMENT OF STATUS EPILEPTICUS IN CHILDREN

Status epilepticus in children is common and has a higher morbidity and mortality than in adults. The same principles of anticonvulsant treatment apply as in adults but dosage adjustments are necessary (Table 8.6).

FURTHER READING

Escueta D *et al*, eds.
Status Epilepticus. New York: Raven Press, 1983. (Advances in Neurology; vol 34).
This comprehensive volume covers most aspects of the subject.

9. Acute Respiratory Failure Due to Neurological Disease

Occasionally, a neurological disorder causing acute respiratory failure presents as a medical emergency although this is much less common than respiratory failure due to primary cardiorespiratory disease. The respiratory failure is due to diaphragmatic and intercostal muscle weakness or paralysis, and the approach to treatment is very different from that in cardiorespiratory disease. Fortunately, the two are easily differentiated in most cases.

The neurological causes of respiratory failure are listed in Table 9.1. Of these, acute peripheral neuropathy (e.g. Guillain-Barré), myasthenia gravis, trauma, coma and, in some countries, acute poliomyelitis are the most important. Respiratory failure in many of the other conditions is rare.

DIAGNOSIS

RESPIRATORY FAILURE
The respiratory failure itself may cause drowsiness, confusion, irritability, restlessness, tachycardia, tachypnoea, a flapping tremor or myoclonic jerking. There will be cyanosis and a poor respiratory excursion. In diaphragmatic paralysis there may be paradoxical respiratory movements with abdominal expansion on expiration — a very useful clinical sign. Auscultation of the chest and heart will be normal in the absence of co-existent pulmonary or cardiac disease.

UNDERLYING NEUROLOGICAL DISEASE
A previous history of neurological disease is often present

Table 9.1 Neurological causes of acute respiratory failure

Central nervous system (e.g. brain stem, anterior horn, spinal cord)	Peripheral nervous system	Neuromuscular junction	Muscle
Coma, from any cause (Chapter 1)	Acute postinfective peripheral neuropathy (e.g. Guillain-Barre)	Myasthenia gravis	Acute myopathy
Trauma (Chapter 6)	Other acute neuropathies†	Myasthenic crisis	Acute deterioration of chronic myopathy/dystrophy
Infection*	Toxic neuropathy‡	Toxins§	Acid maltase deficiency
Stroke (chapter 5)			Carnitine deficiency
Motor neuron disease			Myotonic dystrophy
Acute deterioration of brain-stem, cervical cord lesion			

* e.g. acute poliomyelitis, acute encephalitis, myelitis, encephalomyelitis.
† e.g. diptheria, porphyria.
‡ e.g. thallium poisoning.
§ e.g. botulism, organophosphorous poisoning.

and even where this is not the case a neurological examination may be all that is needed to make a diagnosis. To establish a diagnosis is important, as in some conditions artificial respiration may be inappropriate even in the presence of respiratory failure (e.g. some cases of motor neuron disease). Weakness of the respiratory muscles is seldom the only weakness (exceptions include occasional cases of Guillain-Barré syndrome, polio, acid maltase deficiency and other rare congenital myopathies) and the pattern of truncal and limb muscle weakness, the state of the tendon reflexes and any sensory involvement should allow the diagnosis to be made on clinical grounds in most cases.

In *bulbar disease* there is often an associated dysarthria, a poor cough and dysphagia. In *spinal cord damage* the level must be at C3 or above (the innervation of the diaphragm is C2-C4) and there is usually a severe quadriparesis. In *anterior horn cell disease* there may be wasting, fasciculation and signs of a bulbar palsy. In *acute poliomyelitis* (rare in the UK but commmon in other parts of the world) there may be profound, rapidly progressive limb weakness with preserved sensation, although a pure bulbar syndrome without limb weakness occurs occasionally. If the weakness is due to *peripheral neuropathy*, there is often hyporeflexia and sensory involvement; usually the weakness is most marked distally. In the *Guillain-Barré syndrome*, however, there may sometimes be marked proximal weakness or, indeed, only weakness of the head or neck musculature. In *primary muscle disease* the pattern of weakness is usually symmetrical and may be selective (as in the dystrophies) or proximal (as in the myopathies); there may be other features, such as an associated scoliosis or foot deformities. In *myasthenia gravis* there is usually weakness of the oculomotor and facial muscles and sometimes weakness of the limbs. Differentiation from cardiorespiratory disease is also aided by the absence of a history or specific features of cardiac or pulmonary disorder. Acute respiratory failure may develop in established chronic neurological disease due to super-added aspiration, infection, pulmonary embolism or cardiac involvement.

EMERGENCY MANAGEMENT

IMMEDIATE ASSESSMENT OF VENTILATION

An immediate assessment of ventilation should be made. In the context of neuromuscular or central respiratory failure, assisted ventilation should be instituted if there are clinical signs of respiratory distress; there is significant hypoxia or hypercapnoea; the vital capacity is <1 l/min; inability to cough; or there are signs of progressive neurological deterioration or respiratory exhaustion. Blood gases also may be difficult to evaluate in the presence of chronic respiratory disease.

An endotracheal tube (either nasal or oral) should be inserted and the patient transferred to an intensive care unit where intermittent positive-pressure respiration (or other methods of respiratory assistance) can be arranged. In the absence of co-existent lung or cardiac disease artificial ventilation is usually technically easy and a rapid return of blood chemistry and reversal of symptoms should be expected. The endotracheal tube has the great advantage over external forms of artificial ventilation of preventing inhalation, which is a serious risk in a patient with bulbar weakness. It is important to remember that in acute neuromuscular disease patients needing artificial ventilation are often fully conscious and alert but unable to communicate. Continual reassurance is therefore essential. a few days should be continued via a tracheostomy. Blood gases and biochemistry should be monitored daily. Normally, an anaesthetist should be asked to monitor respiratory function.

If respiratory function is impaired but sufficient to avoid artificial assistance it is usually necessary to admit the patient to an intensive care unit where respiration can be carefully monitored (with FVC measures, not peak flow readings which may not be sufficient). This is especially important if respiratory function is critically impaired or if the neurological condition is fluctuating (e.g. in myasthenia gravis) or progressive (e.g. in Guillain-Barré syndrome).

OTHER MEASURES

A nasogastric tube should be used in cases with associated dysphagia. If the limbs are paralysed, normal skin and nursing care are important and bladder catheterization may be necessary in bulbar or spinal cord disease. Physiotherapy may be vital in controlling infection and the retention of respiratory secretions.

INVESTIGATIONS

A chest X-ray and ECG should be made but will be normal in the absence of co-existent cardiorespiratory disease or inhalation. The blood gases show hypoxia and hypercapnia, and vital capacity and tidal volumes will be reduced. Special investigations depend on the clinical situation but in all cases emergency treatment of the respiratory failure may be needed first. Investigations may include a CSF examination in Guillain-Barré syndrome and poliomyelitis, and an EMG in acute polyneuritis or myopathy. An edrophonium (Tensilon) test may be diagnostic of myasthenia gravis but if respiration is critically impaired it should be carried out in an intensive care unit. The special investigations should be undertaken only after the airway has been protected and adequate respiration established.

10. Brain Death

The development of artificial methods for supporting a patient's circulation and ventilation almost indefinitely has led to the man-made and much debated problem of defining 'brain death' (irreversible cessation of cerebral function). This is important, first, to prevent the prolongation of distressing and pointless treatment, and secondly, because of the possibility of using organs for transplantation. If organ donation is being considered, the transplant team should be alerted before tests to establish brain death are instituted, and the patient's relatives involved at this stage. The following criteria should be all fulfilled before diagnosing brain death.

AETIOLOGY

Aetiology of coma should be established to avoid overlooking the complicating effects of sedative drug overdose or failure to diagnose a potentially treatable condition.

EVALUATION OF CLINICAL NEUROLOGICAL STATUS

* There should be no motor response of any sort.
* The pupils should be fixed and dilated (>3 mm).
* There should be no reflex eye movements (on doll's-head or ice-cold caloric stimulation).
* The corneal and gag reflexes should be absent.
* Spontaneous respiration should be shown to be absent with full carbon dioxide drive. To ensure this and to avoid hypoxia, the patient should be ventilated with 95% oxygen and 5% carbon dioxide for 5 minutes before switching off the ventilator. Then, during the test period, 100% oxygen

Brain Damage

should be given through a tracheal catheter (6–12 l/min). These assessments may be complicated by the presence of severe respiratory disease or chest trauma.

There may occasionally be slight evidence of tendon reflex activity (especially in the legs) and spinal reflex movement in brain-dead patients. If such activity is at all prominent, however, it is safer not to diagnose brain death. Decerebrate or decorticate posturing or seizures do not occur in brain death. The clinical evaluation should always be carried out twice, 24 hours or more apart, by different independent physicians with at least 5 years postgraduate training.

EEG

Although not considered essential by some authorities, it is advisable to confirm death by use of EEG. Two EEGs should be carried out at an interval of more than 24 hours, in which the tracings are both flat (showing no cerebral activity). The gain should be maximized (10–25 v/cm), electrode resistance should be low, and all artefacts

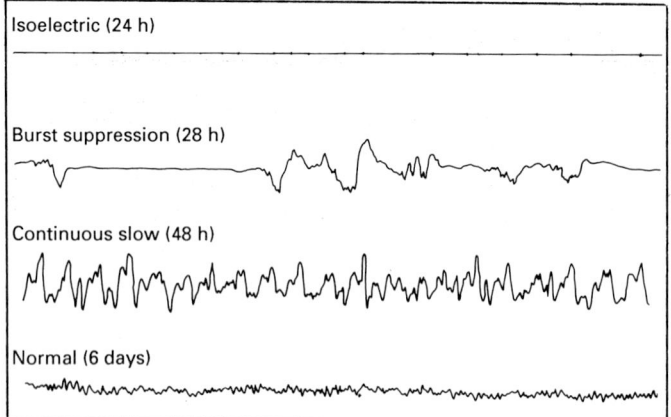

Figure 10. Serial 1 EEG tracing showing acivity after a barbituate overdose. The first EEG is isoelectric and may be mistaken for brain death. Burst suppression is characteristic of barbiturate overdose. The EEG was normal and the patient conscious by the sixth day.

identified and minimized (e.g. those from intensive care instrumentation).

OTHER

The following facts also need to be established before pronouncing brain death.
* That eye drops or systemic drugs that might affect pupillary action (e.g. atropine, morphia) at the time of examination have not been administered.
* That no sedative drugs have been administered or taken that might render the EEG isoelectric (Fig. 10.1). The EEG may remain isoelectric for at least 48 hours following a barbiturate overdose. In cases of sedative drug overdose, it is therefore imperative to wait for a prolonged period before diagnosing brain death.
* That body temperature is adequate, since hypothermia can affect the EEG.
* That no muscle relaxants have been given that could contribute to muscle paralysis at the time of the examination. These drugs should have been stopped at least 48 hours before assessment.

FURTHER READING

Pallis C.
The ABC of Brain Stem Death. London: British Medical Association, 1983.
This collection of articles, published initially in the *British Medical Journal*, covers most aspects of brain death.

Index

Page numbers in *italics* refer to Figures.
Letter *t* after page numbers refer to Tables

abscess, *see* cerebral abscess; spinal epidural abscess; intracranial abscess; subdural empyema
acid-base disturbances, coma 13
acyclovir 23
ADH secretion, inappropriate 69
AIDS encephalitis 22
alcohol
  coma and 4*t*, 6
  head injury and 63
alcoholism 12, 84
amnesia, post-traumatic 63
amphotericin B 38
ampicillin 27*t*, 31*t*
anterior horn cell disease, and respiratory failure 97
antibiotic therapy
  bacterial meningitis 27*t*, 30–36
  cerebral abscess 43
  head injury 64, 66
anticoagulants 47, 55
anticonvulsant therapy
  cerebral abscess 42
  encephalitis 21*t*, 29
  head injury 64, 66, 68, 69
  meningitis 32
  status epilepticus 86–92
    children 93*t*, 94
    intramuscular 92
    long-term 91
    refractory 92–3
  stroke 56
  venous thrombosis/thrombophlebitis 47
antihypertensive agents 55–6
apneustic breathing 8, *9*
ataxic breathing *9*

barbiturate overdose *101*, 102
benzylpenicillin 27*t*, 31*t*
bladder dysfunction 72
blood culture
  cerebral abscess 42
  cerebral venous thrombophlebitis 47
  intracranial subdural empyema 43
  meningitis 32
  stroke 33
brain biopsy 21
brain death 101–3
  aetiology 101
  clinical neurological evaluation 101–2
  EEG 102, *103*
  other 103
bulbar disease, and respiratory failure 97

carbenicillin 31*t*
carcinomatous meningitis 35
carotid angiography, in stroke 54, 56
carotid endarterectomy, in stroke 56
cavernous sinus thrombosis/thrombophlebitis 46–47
cefuroxime 31*t*
cerebral abscess 39–43
  causes 39–40
  clinical features 40–1
  emergency treatment 42–3
  investigations 27*t*, 41–2
cerebral angiography
  cerebral venous thrombosis/thrombophlebitis 47

cerebral angiography (*cont.*)
   intracranial abscess 42, 43
   stroke 54, 56
   subarachnoid haemorrhage 58
cerebral arteries, syndromes of
   51–2, 52*t*
cerebral haemorrhage, *see* stroke
cerebral infarction, *see* stroke
cerebral veins/venous sinuses *44*
cerebral venous thrombosis/
   thrombophlebitis 45–7
   diagnosis 46
   emergency treatment 47
   investigations 46–7
cerebrospinal fluid, *see* CSF
cervical spondylosis 76, 77–8
Cheyne-Strokes respiration 8, *9*
children, status epilepticus 93*t*,
   94
chloramphenicol 27*t*, 31*t*, 36
chlormethiazole, status
   epilepticus 88*t*, 90, 93*t*
cluster breathing *9*
coma 1–17
   causes 2–6, 34
   diffuse neurological or
      systemic disorders 3–4*t*,
      5–6
   emergency investigations 11*t*
   emergency resuscitation 6
   emergency treatment 12–14
   eye movements in 9–10
   focal subtentorial lesions 3*t*,
      4–5
   focal supratentorial lesions 3*t*,4
   Glasgow Coma Scale 2*t*, 7–8
   initial diagnostic assessment
      6–11
   level of consciousness in 7–8
   position *6*
   pupillary reactions in 8–9
   serial monitoring 1, 2, 11–12,
      64
   transtentorial herniation
      (coning) 14–17
   see also brain death; head injury
conjugate eye movement 5, 9, 10
consciousness, level of 7–8
cortical vein thrombosis/
   thrombophlebitis 45, 46*t*
corticosteroids
   acute encephalitis 22, 23

corticosteroids (*cont.*)
   bacterial meningitis 33
   cerebral abscess 42
   coma 12, 15
   intracerebral haemorrhage 68
   spinal cord compression 79, 81
   see also dexamethasone
cranial nerve injury 69
cranial nerve palsies 11
CSF examination and lumbar
   puncture 27*t*
   cerebral abscess 27*t*, 42, 43
   cerebral venous thrombosis/
      thrombophlebitis 47
   coma 15, 11*t*
   encephalitis 20, 21, 22, 27*t*
   extradural abscess 27*t*, 45
   head injury 62*t*
   meningitis 26, 27*t*, 29, 30, 33,
      34, 35, 36, 37, 38
   non compressive spinal cord
      disease 79
   status epilepticus 85
   stroke 51, 55
   subarachnoid haemorrhage 57
   subdural empyema 27*t*, 43
   supratentorial mass lesions 15
CT scanning (computed
   tomography)
   cerebral abscess 41
   cerebral venous thrombosis/
      thrombophlebitis 47
   coma 11*t*, 5, 14
   encephalitis 21
   head injury 67, 68, 69
   intracranial extradural abscess
      45
   intracranial subdural empyema
      43
   meningitis 33
   status epilepticus 85
   stroke 51, 54
   subarachnoid haemorrhage 57

decerebrate movements 10, 102
decorticate movements 10, 102
dexamethasone 12, 15, 22, 23, 42,
   47, 79, 81
   see also corticosteroids
diabetic coma 1, 4*t*, 6
diaphragmatic paralysis 95

diazepam, status epilepticus 86–7, 88t, 93t
disc disease, spinal compression 75–6

edrophonium (Tensilon) test 99
EEG (electroencephalogram)
  acute viral encephalitis 21
  brain death 102, 103
  cerebral abscess 42
  coma 5, 11t
  status epilepticus 92
encephalitis, infective 19–23
  acute viral 19–23, 27t
    causes 20t
    clinical features 19–20, 20t
    diagnosis 20–2
    emergency treatment 22–3
  non-viral 23
  post-viral 19
encephalomyelitis, postviral 19
epidural (extradural) abscess
  intracranial 27t, 39, 44–5
  spinal 75
epidural (extradural) haematoma, spinal 76
epidural (extradural) haemorrhage, intracranial 66–7
epilepsy
  status epilepticus in 83, 85, 86t
  see also seizures
extradural haemorrhage, acute in head injury 3t, 66–7
eye movements, reflex 9–10, 101

flucloxacillin 31t
flucytosine 38
fungal meningitis 27t, 35, 37–8

gentamicin 27t, 31t
Glasgow Coma Scale 1, 7, 8t, 10
glucose infusion 12, 84
Guillain-Barré syndrome, and respiratory failure 97

head injury 61–70
  admission to hospital 63t, 63
  early hospital management 64–5
  immediate complications 65, 70
  initial assessment 61–2

head injury (*cont.*)
  open 65
  skull X-ray, criteria for 62t
  transfer to neurological unit 65
herpes simplex encephalitis 19, 21, 23
Herxheimer reaction, in neurosyphilis 32
hypertension, stroke 55–6
hyperthermia 13
hyperventilation, forced 12, 17
hypoglycaemia 12, 84
hypotension
  coma 7
  spinal cord injury 81
hypothermia 13, 103
hypoxia, status epilepticus 93

infections
  acute intracranial 19t
  coma 13
  spinal 75
  see also cerebral abscess;
    cortical vein thrombosis/thrombophlebitis;
    encephalitis, infective;
    meningitis; subdural empyema
internal carotid artery occlusion 52
intracerebral haematoma 58
intracerebral haemorrhage
  acute in head injury 3t, 68–9
  acute traumatic 68–9
  differentiation from stroke 50–1
intracranial abscess 39–45
  see also cerebral abscess;
    extradural abscess;
    subdural empyema
intracranial infections, classification 19t
intracranial pressure, raised
  acute encephalitis 22
  bacterial meningitis 33–4
  coma 12
intramuscular anticonvulsant therapy 92

lacerations, scalp 62, 65
lumbar puncture, *see* CSF examination

mannitol 12, 17, 68
meningitis 25–38
  bacterial 28–37
    acute complications 33t
    antibiotic treatment 27t, 30–2, 36
    causes 28t, 29t
    clinical features 28–9
    diagnostic and management problems 33–7
    emergency investigations 30t
    emergency treatment 30–2
    focal neurological signs/coma 34
    laboratory findings 27t, 29–30
    optic disc changes 33–4
    partially treated 34
  carcinomatous 35
  clinical features 25–6
  fungal 27t, 35, 37–8
  neonatal 36–7
  parasitic 38
  recurrent 35–6
  sterile 34–5, 38
  symptoms and signs 25t
  tuberculous 27t, 35, 37
  viral 25–7, 35
    laboratory findings 26, 27t
    treatment 26
meningo-encephalitis 20
meningovascular syphilis 38
metabolic disturbances
  coma 5, 13
  status epilepticus 93
motor function, comatose patients 10–11
motor weakness
  respiratory failure 97
  spinal cord dysfunction 71–2
muscle disease, primary and respiratory function 97
muscle relaxants 103
myasthenia gravis, and respiratory function 97, 99
myelitis, acute transverse 76, 79
myelography 78–9

naloxone 13
neonatal meningitis 36–7

oculocephalic reflex 9–10

oculovestibular reflex 9–10
optic disc changes, bacterial meningitis 33–4
overdose, drug and coma 4t, 6

papilloedema 4, 11, 33
paraldehyde, status epilepticus 88t, 91, 93t
penicillin 27t, 31t, 38
peripheral neuropathy, respiratory failure 97
phenytoin
  head injury 64
  intramuscular 92
  status epilepticus 87–90, 91, 93t
poliomyelitis, acute and respiratory failure 97
poliovirus 25
prednisone, in Herxheimer reaction 38
pseudoseizures 83, 93
pupillary reactions 8–9, 101, 103

respiratory failure 73, 95–9
  brain death 101–2
  diagnosis 95
  emergency management 98–9
  investigations 99
  neurological causes 95–7
respiratory function, assessment 98–9
respiratory patterns, coma 8, 9

scalp lacerations 62, 65
seizures
  bacterial meningitis 32t
  coma 5, 13
  encephalitis 21t, 29
  meningitis 32
  post-traumatic 69
  stroke 56
  venous thrombosis/thrombophlebitis 47
  see also status epilepticus
sensory disturbances, spinal disease 72, 73
skull fracture
  cerebral abscess 39
  depressed 66
  diagnosis 62
  linear 66
  recurrent meningitis 36

Index

sphincteric dysfunction 72
spinal column, degenerative
    disease 76
spinal cord, vascular infarction
    76–7
spinal cord dysfunction 71–81
    acute compression 74t, 74–6,
        78–9
    acute non-compressive lesions
        76–8, 79
    clinical features 71–3
    emergency management 78–9
    respiratory failure 73, 97
spinal cord injury 79–81
    emergency assessment 80
    movement of patient 80
    other injuries 81
    radiological diagnosis 80–1
    treatment 81
spinal epidural abscess 75
spinal epidural haematoma 76
spinal pain 71
spinal tumours
    metastatic 74–5
    primary 75
spondylosis 76
status epilepticus 83–94
    aetiology and precipitating
        factors 85
    anticonvulsant therapy 86–92
    children 93t, 94
    emergency investigations 84–5
    emergency management 84
    medical complications 85, 86t
    refractory 92–3
stroke 49–56
    causes 52–3, 53t
    clinical features 52t

stroke (*cont.*)
    diagnosis 49–53
        differentiation of infarction
            and haemorrhage 50–1
        localization of site of damage
            51–2
    differential diagnosis 50t
    emergency investigations 53–5
    emergency management 55–6
subarachnoid haemorrhage 57–9
    diagnosis 57
    emergency investigations 57
    emergency management 58–9
subdural abscess 27t
subdural empyema 39, 43–4
subdural haemorrhage
    acute in head injury 3t, 66–7
    acute traumatic 67–8
subhyaloid retinal haemorrhage
    11, 57
subtentorial lesions 3t, 4–5
supratentorial lesions 1, 3t, 4, 14–17
syphilis, meningovascular 38

thiamine 12, 84
thiopentone, refractory status
    epilepticus 92
transtentorial herniation (coning)
    1, 13, 14–17, 42, 66–7
transverse myelitis, acute 76, 79
tuberculous meningitis 27t, 35, 37

uncal herniation 14, *15*

vaccination, encephalomyelitis
    and 18
ventilation, assisted 84, 98
vertebral artery occlusion 52t